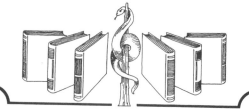

CLINICAL ATLAS
OF
AUDITORY EVOKED POTENTIALS

CLINICAL ATLAS OF AUDITORY EVOKED POTENTIALS

Edited by

Jeffrey H. Owen, Ph.D.

Assistant Research Professor
Division of Orthopedic Surgery
Department of Surgery
Washington University School of Medicine
St. Louis, Missouri

Charles D. Donohoe, M.D.

Associate Clinical Professor of Neurology
Kansas University Medical Center
Kansas City, Kansas

Grune & Stratton, Inc.
Harcourt Brace Jovanovich Publishers

Orlando   New York   San Diego   London
San Francisco   Tokyo   Sydney   Toronto

Grune & Stratton, Inc.
Orlando, Florida 32887

Distributed in the United Kingdom by
Grune & Stratton, Ltd.
24/28 Oval Road, London NW 1

Library of Congress Catalog Number 87-082754
International Standard Book Number 0-8089-1896-6
Printed in the United States of America
87 88 89 90   10 9 8 7 6 5 4 3 2 1

This text is dedicated to Hallowell Davis, M.D. Starting at Harvard University and continuing through his position at Central Institute for the Deaf, Dr. Davis has provided a stimulating guidance to the field of electrophysiology, especially in the area of electric response audiometry. As a professional mentor, I have been privileged to work with him; as a personal friend I have had the rare opportunity to experience an enlightened individual.

Contents

Preface

During the last 40 years, the progress in neurologic diagnosis in large measure has paralleled advances in neuroradiologic technology. Cerebral angiography, myelography, computed tomography, and magnetic resonance have directed the methodology and set standards in clinical neurology. These advances in technique have made conventional neuropathologic diagnoses more easily accessible. Therapeutic strides have tended to follow a similar course.

With the advent of neurochemistry, neuroimmunology, and neurophysiology, the technology serves not only to confirm clinical impressions but to define, quantify, and reshape our understanding of a disorder. Realizing that the microcomputer and its application in clinical neurophysiology is in its inception, the ability to expand on the physiologic aspects of the clinical exam represents a worthy goal. During the current embryonic stage of this process, abuses and unrealistic expectations can be anticipated. Ultimately, we feel that the final result will make neurology a more objective and decisive discipline. Techniques derived from these preliminary procedures will eventually filter into the office of the practicing physician and enlighten our perceptions of neurologic illness. We also expect, as the clinical neurologic method becomes more precise, the very relationship between patient and doctor will assume a more humane and honest climate.

As editors of this volume, we sincerely thank all contributors. We commend their hardwork and personally appreciate their unselfish willingness to participate. We have all found that the evaluation of technology can be as complex as its development. Although the future holds promise for evoked potentials, the field cannot be sustained purely by hope; broadened practical applicability is needed.

Contributors

Charles D. Donohoe, M.D.
Associate Clinical Professor of Neurology, Kansas
University Medical Center, Kansas City, Kansas

John A. Ferraro, Ph.D.
Professor and Chairman, Department of Hearing and
Speech; Associate Dean, School of Allied Health,
University of Kansas Medical Center, Kansas City, Kansas

James W. Hall III, Ph.D
Associate Professor and Chief of Audiology, Department of
Otolaryngology–Head and Neck Surgery, University of
Texas Medical School; Director of Audiology, Hermann
Hospital, Houston, Texas

Robert Aaron Levine, M.D.
Eaton-Peabody Laboratory, Massachusetts Eye and Ear
Infirmary, Boston, Massachusetts

Jeffrey H. Owen, Ph.D.
Assistant Research Professor, Division of Orthopedic
Surgery, Department of Surgery, Washington University
School of Medicine, St. Louis, Missouri

Louise D. Resor, M.D.
Neurologist, Director of Electroencephalography, Stanford
Hospital, Stanford, Connecticut

Denise A. Tucker, M.CD.
Audiologist, Department of Pediatrics, Texas Tech Health
Sciences Center, Amarillo, Texas

John A. Ferraro

1
Electrocochleography

Electrocochleography (ECochG) has become an important tool in the identification, assessment, and monitoring of certain otological and audiological disorders. In general, ECochG is a method of recording the stimulus-related potentials of the peripheral auditory system. The specific responses recorded may include the cochlear microphonic (CM) and components of the summating potential (SP) of the cochlea, and the whole-nerve or compound action potential (AP) of the auditory nerve.

It is generally acknowledged that the first recording of human CM was reported by Fromm et al. in 1935, although several features of both the CM and the auditory nerve AP had been described based on animal studies before this time. By 1950, the CM had been recorded by numerous other investigators using electrodes on or near the round window of subjects undergoing ear surgery (Andreev et al., 1939; Perlman and Case, 1941; Lempert et al., 1947; Lempert et al., 1950). The human auditory nerve AP was first recorded by Ruben and his co-workers in 1960, also during ear surgery.

Perhaps the most significant factor in the development of clinical ECochG to the current era was the application of signal-averaging techniques, which allowed for nonsurgical recordings (Ronis, 1966). Yoshie et al. (1967) initiated extratympanic recordings using subdermal, ear canal electrodes, whereas Portmann and Aran (1972) utilized a transtympanic approach with the primary electrode seated on the promontory.

In the 1970s, ECochG received comparatively little attention as a clinical tool, especially in the United States. Recently, however, there has been a renewed interest in the clinical application of this technique, and many laboratories and clinics engaged in evoked response testing are beginning to utilize ECochG once again.

Several reasons account for the gaining popularity of clinical ECochG; the widespread application and acceptance of auditory evoked response testing in general, and of the auditory brainstem response (ABR) in particular, are certainly among these. In addition, technological advancements and improvements in recording systems have made these very early responses easier to extract using noninvasive, extratympanic techniques. This eliminates pain or discomfort to the patient as well as the need for anesthetics. Furthermore, a physician does not have to be present to insert the primary electrode and to monitor the status of the patient during the recording session. Perhaps the most important reason for the renewed attention to ECochG is, however, that the information obtained from an examination can be very helpful to the physician in the diagnosis and treatment of certain audiological and otological disorders, especially Meniere's disease and endolymphatic hydrops (MD/ELH).

Given the current status of clinical ECochG and the role that recording methodology has played in renewing interest in this area, the information presented in this chapter will pertain to the use of noninvasive, extratympanic recording techniques. The material is organized to include: a summarization of the salient features of the CM, SP, and AP as the responses being recorded; a description of our recording techniques (electrodes, parameters of stimulation, and response acquisition); definitions of normal and clinically abnormal response characteristics; and case studies from our laboratory wherein ECochG was part of the examination battery.

Clinical Atlas of Auditory Evoked Potentials
ISBN 0-8089-1896-6

AUDITORY STIMULUS-RELATED RESPONSES

COCHLEAR MICROPHONIC

The CM was discovered by Wever and Bray in 1930, and, at least in animals, has probably been the most thoroughly investigated potential of the inner ear. This historical popularity is due in part to the relative magnitude of the response (which is large) and the ease with which it can be recorded.

As opposed to the "resting" potentials of the cochlea, the CM is clearly stimulus-related and "duplicates to a great extent the displacement-time pattern of the cochlear partition." (Dallos, 1973, p. 24). Appearing as an alternating current (AC) voltage, the CM will mirror the waveform of low to moderately intense acoustic stimuli. When recorded from a normal ear with the primary electrode seated in the middle ear (i.e., promontory or round window), the CM output stems primarily from the cochlear generators within a few millimeters of the electrode, specifically, the outer hair cells of the basal turn (Dallos, 1973). When the electrode is in the ear canal, the distance from the generators is uniform, providing for a more general but less sensitive picture of cochlear function (Elberling and Salomon, 1973). Whether the CM has an actual role in transduction at the hair cell level or is merely an epiphenomenon of the process is still a disputed issue.

As mentioned earlier, CM has been recorded in man by both surgical and nonsurgical methods. Elberling and Salomon (1973), for example, used an averaging technique to record CM from the ear canal in both normally and abnormally hearing individuals. The primary manifestation of cochlear pathology seen in the CM was a reduction in response magnitude. Other investigators (Morrison et al., 1980; Moriuchi and Kumagami, 1979; Kumagami et al., 1982) have reported reduced CM magnitudes and waveform distortion in patients suffering from Meniere's disease. Gibson and Beagley (1976) and Morrison et al. (1980) have even observed a "prolonged after ringing" of the CM in the early stages of endolymphatic hydrops. It has been our experience that the response variability associated with the CM in both normal and abnormal ears, and the difficulty encountered in accurately interpreting CM findings, make this particular potential less applicable than others for clinical ECochG, especially in the diagnosis of MD/ELH. More recently, Gerhardt et al. (1985) have combined ECochG and ABR findings in the diagnosis of acoustic neuromas. Their diagnostic criteria for tumors included an increased latency of the auditory nerve AP and a low amplitude ratio between the AP and the CM. The reader is referred to this article for a more detailed description of CM recording techniques and current application in ECochG.

SUMMATING POTENTIAL

The SP was identified by Davis and his colleagues and independently by von Bekesy in the early 1950s (Davis et al, 1950; von Bekesy, 1950). Current evidence regarding the properties and role of this particular potential(s), however, is inconclusive. This is certainly due in part to the complexity of the response, which comprises several components, and the measurement of which is affected by an interaction between stimulus parameters and electrode location.

Like the CM, the SP is also stimulus-related, arising from the hair cells of the organ of Corti. Unlike the CM, however, the SP is seen as a direct current (DC) voltage that, at least to some degree, represents the envelope of the evoking stimulus (Dallos, 1973). The polarity of the DC shift may be positive or negative, depending on the frequency and intensity of the acoustic stimulus, and the location of the recording electrodes. Using conventional extratympanic ECochG recording techniques, the SP from a normal ear appears to be dominated by the Differential (DIF)-component (Dallos et al., 1972). This is characterized by a negative shift in the baseline of the recorded response, which persists for the duration of the evoking stimulus. The DC response to an AC stimulus identifies the SP as a distortion product. This implies that at least some of the SP components are representative of cochlear mechanical or mechano-electrical nonlinearity (Tasaki et al., 1954; Whitfield and Ross, 1965).

Several studies have now shown that the ECochG response recorded from patients suspected of having MD/ELH is often characterized by an enlarged summating potential component (e.g., Schmidt et al., 1974; Gibson et al., 1977; Kitahara et al., 1981; Coats, 1981; Goin et al., 1982; Ferraro et al., 1983; Ferraro et al., 1985). The rationale generally proposed for this finding is that the presence of endolymphatic hydrops will alter the hydromechanical properties of the inner ear due to an increase in endolymph volume and intralabyrinthine pressure. When this occurs, the normal vibratory asymmetry of the basilar membrane will be augmented. This increased distortion within the system, in turn, will be reflected by an increase in the magnitude of the SP. Another perspective is that hydrops will create an additional "bias" on the membrane analagous to that observed by Durrant and Dallos (1972), and Durrant and Gans (1977), when they electrically biased the system and observed enlarged SPs. Support for these hypotheses is indirect at best and virtually impossible to verify in humans at the present time. Goin et al. (1982) have suggested that other factors, such as biochemical and/or vascular changes, may also play a role. Regardless of specific pathophysiology, however, an enlarged SP does appear to be associated with MD/ELH, and is rarely observed when hydrops can definitely be ruled out.

AUDITORY NERVE ACTION POTENTIAL

The whole-nerve or compound AP of the auditory nerve has been the most popular ECochG component studied in humans (Ruben et al., 1960; Sohmer and Feinmesser, 1967; Coats and Dickey, 1970; Cullen et al., 1972). Until recently, in fact, it was generally assumed that the term electrocochleography referred primarily to the recording of the auditory nerve AP. Recordable from several sites (e.g., directly from the nerve; round window, promontory; tympanic membrane; ear canal), the AP represents the summed response of several thousand individual nerve fibers that have fired in synchrony. The response to click stimuli is generally referred to as "whole-nerve" AP and suggests that neural activity from the entire length of the basilar membrane is represented. The term "compound" AP is used when the evoking stimuli are tone bursts, and implies that a more limited segment of the basilar membrane contributes to the response (Gibson, 1978). This terminology is somewhat misleading in that the synchronous activity essential for producing the AP is seen at the onset of a tone-burst or in response to clicks. Kiang (1965), in turn, has shown that this onset response is dominated by neural contributions from the basal, high-frequency end of the cochlea.

Like the CM (but unlike the SP), the AP is also seen as an AC voltage, and is generally characterized by a short series of brief, predominantly negative peaks. The first and primary component of the AP is negative and usually referred to as N_1. This is virtually the same component as Wave I of the ABR (Jewett and Williston, 1971). Both the magnitude and latency of N_1 are dependent on the intensity of the evoking stimulus. For practical purposes, we can define latency as the time between the onset of the electrical signal that drives the acoustic transducer and the N_1 peak. AP magnitude reflects the number of fibers firing, while N_1 latency is a reflection of stimulus travel time, propagation time along the basilar membrane, and the time associated with the synchronization of the neural responses that contribute to the peak. In general, as stimulus intensity is decreased from suprathreshold levels, AP magnitude decreases and N_1 latency increases.

For clinical purposes it may be feasible, in some cases, to compare AP (N_1) thresholds with behavioral thresholds to the evoking stimulus. Indeed, the earlier applications of ECochG were aimed at identifying/confirming hearing loss in difficult-to-test populations (e.g., children) (Cullen et al., 1972). With noninvasive, extratympanic techniques, however, this has not proven to be particularly useful, especially in comparison to the utility of Wave V of the ABR for this purpose.

As discussed previously, the ECochG waveform recorded from patients suspected of having MD/ELH is often characterized by an enlarged SP. The clinical consistency of this finding, however, appears to improve when the SP amplitude is compared to the AP amplitude (Coats, 1981; Kitahara et al., 1981; Goin et al., 1982; Gibbin et al., 1983; Ferraro et al., 1983, 1985; Ferraro and Ruth, 1985). There is a tendency for the SP:AP amplitude ratio to be considerably enlarged in the suspected presence of endolymphatic hydrops.

EXTRATYMPANIC RECORDING TECHNIQUES

Currently, it appears that the most popular and clinically relevant application of extratympanic (ET) ECochG is in the diagnosis, assessment, and monitoring of MD/ELH. When recorded for this purpose, the response consists of a complex waveform containing both SP and AP components. ET recording techniques and parameters are therefore designed to extract these particular auditory stimulus-related potentials.

RECORDING ELECTRODES

There has been a variety of primary electrode types used to record ET ECochG. Examples include an earlobe clip (Sohmer and Feinmesser, 1967), a ball-tipped silver wire against the skin

of the ear canal or on the tympanic membrane (Cullen et al., 1972), and a foam rubber earplug with silver wire mounted on its surface (Yanz and Dodds, 1985).

Recently, ET recording electrodes have even become commercially available. Perhaps the most popular is a silver-ball, leaf electrode, or "eartrode" developed by Coats (1974) and manufactured by Life-Tech, Inc., of Houston, Texas. The eartrode is composed of dimel-insulated silver wire that leads to a silver ball-tip. Pictured in Figure 1-1 (from Ferraro et al., 1986) the tip and initial portion of the electrode are glued to a strip of mylar plastic. The eartrode is designed to be wedged into the ear canal with the ball-tip held stationary against the skin by pressure from the plastic. We rest the tip in the posterior-inferior quadrant of the canal near the cartilaginous-bony junction.

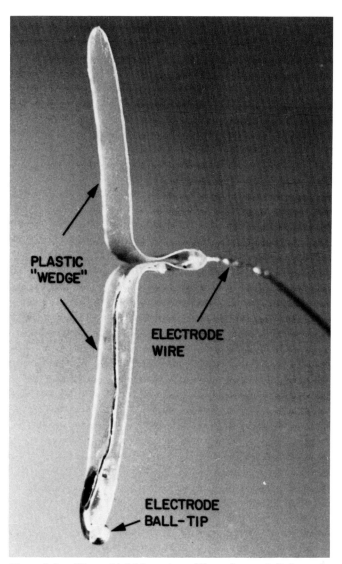

PLASTIC "WEDGE"

ELECTRODE WIRE

ELECTRODE BALL-TIP

Figure 1-1. Tip and initial portion of Coats "eartrode" electrode (Life-Tech Inc., Houston, TX). (Reprinted from Ferraro, JA, & Murphy, GB, & Ruth, RA (1986). A comparative study of primary electrodes used in extratympanic electrocochleography. In JA Ferraro (Ed.), *Electrocochleography, Seminars in Hearing.* New York: Thieme-Stratton. p. 279. With permission.)

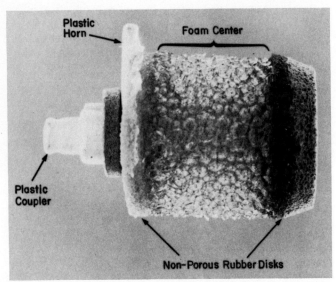

Figure 1-2. 3M earplug electrode (3M Otodiagnostics Systems Inc., St. Paul, MN). (Reprinted from Ferraro, JA, & Murphy, GB, & Ruth, RA (1986). A comparative study of primary electrodes used in extratympanic electrocochleography. In JA Ferraro (Ed.), *Electrocochleography, Seminars in Hearing.* New York: Thieme-Stratton. p. 280. With permission.)

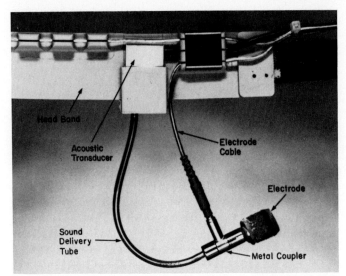

Figure 1-3. 3M earplug electrode attached to headband module. (Reprinted from Ferraro, JA, & Murphy, GB, & Ruth, RA (1986). A comparative study of primary electrodes used in extratympanic electrocochleography. In JA Ferraro (Ed.), *Electrocochleography, Seminars in Hearing.* New York: Thieme-Stratton. p. 280. With permission.)

The magnitude of the response will be larger if the tip is positioned nearer, or at the eardrum (i.e. in comparison to a "shallower" ear canal placement). However, positioning the electrode closer to the eardrum usually creates some discomfort for the patient, increases the risk of traumatizing the eardrum, and may necessitate the assistance of a physician.

More recently, a disposable, foam earplug electrode has also become commercially available (3M Otodiagnostic Systems Inc., St. Paul, Minnesota). Pictured in Figure 1-2 (from Ferraro et al., 1986), the foam earplug consists of front and back disks made of non-porous rubber, and a reticulated foam center saturated with electrode gel. The back disk attaches to a silver-plated plastic horn and coupler that allows for placement consistency and also prevents the earplug from penetrating the ear canal deeply enough to endanger the tympanic membrane. As seen in Figure 1-3 (from Ferraro et al., 1986), the earplug is part of a system that includes a headband module. The plastic coupler of the electrode attaches to this module via a metal coupler that also accepts the sound delivery tube from a miniature acoustic transducer on the headband. The sound delivery tube/channel runs through the center of the earplug.

A study comparing ECochG recordings made with the Life-Tech eartrode, 3M earplug, and a gold-plated disc (surface) electrode over the mastoid process identified the 3M earplug as potentially the most suitable for clinical purposes (Ferraro et al., 1986). In this study, the quality of the responses recorded with the Life-Tech and 3M electrodes was very similar, and superior to that observed in the responses recorded with the mastoid disc electrode. However, the 3M electrode had considerably lower impedances, was easier to place and took less time to place, and was more stable after placement in comparison to the eartrode.

RECORDING PARAMETERS

Table 1-1 illustrates the parameters we currently utilize for ET ECochG. These are very similar to those employed for standard ABR recording, with some notable exceptions. First of all, the electrode montage is such that the primary electrode/recording site is the ear canal of the stimulated ear. The secondary site can be the contralateral ear canal or earlobe or mastoid process, with ground at the forehead. Interchanging of secondary and ground sites appears to have minimal effect on the response

Table 1-1 Recording Parameters

Electrode Montage	
Primary site (voltage positive):	ipsilateral ear canal
Secondary site (voltage negative):	contralateral ear canal/earlobe
Ground:	forehead
Signal Averager Settings	
Repetitions:	1000–2000
Analysis time:	5–10 msec
Amplification:	50,000–100,000X
Filter band-pass:	3–3000Hz
Stimuli	
Type:	broad-band clicks
Duration:	100-μsec electrical pulse
Hearing level:	begin at maximum output (90–95 dB)
Polarity:	alternating
Repetition rate:	9–11/sec

(i.e., the forehead may serve as the secondary site). Using this montage, negative polarity will be displayed in a downward direction.

The number of stimulus repetitions needed to evoke a well-defined response may vary from patient to patient. Generally speaking, however, it has been our experience that 1000–2000 samples is sufficient in virtually all cases.

The response we are attempting to record occurs within the first 3–5 msec after stimulus onset. The analysis time or window, therefore, must allow for a detailed visualization of this very early period. Again based on our experience, 10 msec is suitable. We have even used a 20-msec window and expanded the horizontal time base of our oscilloscope interface to enhance the first 5 msec of electrophysiological activity.

Pre-amplifier amplification factor may be as high as 100,000X. At this high a setting, however, and depending on the level of background electrical and electroencephalographic (EEG) "noise," the artifact rejection mode of the evoked response system may be engaged continuously. If this is the case, an amplification factor of 50,000X is an acceptable compromise. An additional amplification factor may be built into the signal averager and will vary among instruments.

The band-pass of the pre-amplifier filter must be wide enough to allow for the amplification of both a DC (the SP) and an AC (the AP) response. This presents a dilemma, in that we are attempting to amplify a DC response through an AC pre-amplification system. Even though the high-pass cut-off of the filter is very low at 3–10Hz, there will still be some distortion of at least the SP component of the waveform. In essence, when using a standard evoked response system, we are probably recording a distorted reflection of the SP (i.e., a "distorted distortion component"). This presents a limitation to which we have previously called attention (Ferraro et al., 1983, 1985), which should be considered in the interpretation of clinical findings.

Stimuli used to evoke the ECochG responses are generally broad-band clicks. The duration of the electrical pulse from the stimulus generator to the transducer is usually 100 μsec. It is important to note that this is not the duration of the actual acoustic stimulus. The transmission characteristics of the transducer will modify this pulse to produce a longer signal. The relevance of this is apparent when one remembers that the duration of the SP is dependent on the duration of the evoking stimulus.

In order to evoke a well-defined SP-AP complex, we begin stimulus presentation at the maximum dB output of our signal generator (95 dB Hearing Level or HL) at a rate of 9-11/sec. Click polarity is alternated to inhibit the appearance of cochlear microphonic and stimulus artifact. Contralateral masking is unnecessary in that the ECochG responses are generated prior to crossover of the auditory pathway. In addition, the magnitude of any response in the opposite ear to a bone-conducted signal will be too small to interfere with the response from the stimulated ear.

Finally, we have found it extremely useful to continuously monitor background EEG activity on another oscilloscope (i.e., aside from the oscilloscope interface of evoked response system). This allows us to monitor and assess environmental electrical noise and alerts us to potential problems associated with electrode placement and contact, as well as excessive swallowing and/or muscle tension from the patient. In order to do this, the output from the biological pre-amplifier received by the signal averager must also be directed into the monitoring oscilloscope.

RESPONSE CHARACTERISTICS

NORMAL RESPONSE

Figure 1-4 (from Ferraro et al., 1985) displays a normal ET-ECochG response, evoked using the recording parameters identified in Table 1-1. The components or portions of the SP-AP complex routinely analyzed are labeled, and include the duration and amplitude of each component, and the latency of the AP-N_1 peak.

There is variation in the literature regarding how and where the above components/portions are measured. We define the SP as the "shoulder" preceding the onset of the AP-N_1. The duration of the SP as defined in Figure 1-4 may only represent what appears to be the negative component of this potential, as measured from its onset to the onset of the first negative deflection of the AP (i.e., the N_1). Defining duration in this manner, however, has maximized consistency across subjects with respect to this particular parameter. AP duration is measured from the onset of N_1 to the first positive peak following N_1. SP amplitude is measured peak-to-trough, whereas AP amplitude is reflected in the distance between the onset and peak of N_1. It is important to

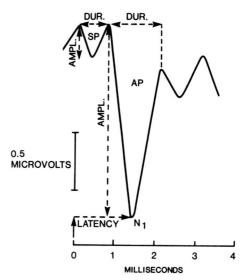

Figure 1-4. Normal click-evoked ECochG waveform. Components and portions measured are labeled. Solid arrow indicates click onset. SP = summating potential; AP = action potential. (Reprinted from Ferraro, JA, & Arenberg, IK, & Hassanein, RS (1985). Electrocochleography and symptoms of inner ear dysfunction. *Arch Otolaryngol, 111*, p. 72. Copyright 1985, American Medical Association. With permission.)

Table 1-2 Normative Data

	Summating Potential		Action Potential			Summating Potential: Action Potential Amplitude ratio
	Duration (msec)	Amplitude (μvolt)	Duration (msec)	Amplitude (μvolt)	N₁ Latency (msec)	
Mean	0.36	0.37	1.04	1.35	1.50	0.28
Range	0.30–0.50	0.10–1.00	0.80–1.25	0.60–3.10	1.30–1.70	0.11–0.47
Standard deviation	0.02	0.20	0.10	0.60	0.10	0.10

note that several investigators measure SP and AP amplitudes with respect to a pre- or post-stimulus baseline. Whether one chooses to make comparative amplitude measurements, or uses a more "absolute" indication as we do, will be reflected in the normative values for these parameters. These established "norms," which are usually specific for a given laboratory or clinic, will be the basis for clinical comparisons. In essence, the normative value of an ECochG parameter will vary across laboratories according to how and where the parameter is defined and measured.

Table 1-2 illustrates the normative values (means, ranges, and standard deviations) from our laboratory for the ECochG components described in the preceding paragraph. As can be seen from this Table, SP duration is a relatively consistent feature, ranging from 0.3–0.5 msec across ears. Once again, this value is a reflection of stimulus duration, and variations across ears may be due in part to acoustic transducer and sound delivery effects. AP duration is very stable within ears, but more variable than is SP duration across ears. Gibson et al. (1977) have observed a widening of the SP-AP complex in Meniere's disease. Gibbin et al. (1983), however, have not found measurement of width (or duration) of the complex to be of clinical value, due to the difficulty in determining when the response returns to baseline. Our findings are in general agreement with Gibbin et al. We have been unable to observe changes in component durations that are consistent and specific enough to associate with a particular pathological condition.

Both SP and AP amplitude show considerable variation across and within ears. This finding has also been reported by others (e.g., Gibbin et al., 1983). What appears to be a more consistent amplitude feature, however, is the percentage amplitude, or amplitude ratio between the SP and AP. Normal values in our laboratory range from approximately 0.10 to 0.50 (i.e., 10–50 percent), with a mean of approximately 0.25, or 25 percent.

AP-N₁ latency will show minimal fluctuation across normal ears. Since N₁ of the AP and Wave I of the ABR are the same component, N₁ and Wave I latencies should be identical if ECochG and ABR are recorded independently to the same stimulus.

ABNORMAL RESPONSE

Figure 1-5 illustrates the ECochG tracings and pure-tone audiograms from 3 different patients. Repeat tracings, which are always recorded, are eliminated from this figure for the sake of simplicity. Data from Patient 1 (top) show that the AP amplitude and N₁ latency of the left response are reduced and delayed, respectively, in comparison to the right amplitude and latency. This is probably a reflection of the slightly greater degree of high-frequency hearing loss in the left ear, as indicated by the corresponding audiogram. The SP:AP amplitude ratio, however, is within normal limits.

ECochG tracings from the left ear of Patient 2 (middle) display reduced, distorted, and delayed components. The presence of the SP, in fact, is questionable. This pattern is consistent with a greater degree of high-frequency, sensorineural hearing loss, as is illustrated in the corresponding audiogram for this patient. In this instance, the SP:AP amplitude ratio appears to be abnormally reduced.

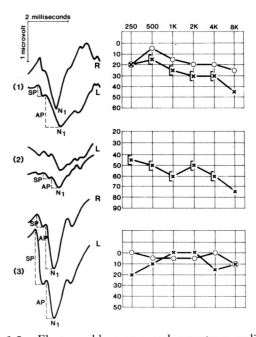

Figure 1-5. Electrocochleograms and pure-tone audiograms from 3 different patients. Top tracings (1) display a reduced and delayed left ECochG response reflective of the slightly greater degree of high-frequency hearing loss in the left ear in comparison to the right ear. Middle tracings (2) display reduced and distorted waveforms reflective of moderate hearing loss. Lower tracings (3) are from a patient with Meniere's disease in the left ear. The right electrocochleogram is normal, whereas the left is characterized by an enlarged SP and SP:AP amplitude ratio.

The lower tracings in Figure 1-5 are from a patient with a brief history of Meniere's disease. The right ECochG response is well within normal limits, but the left tracing is characterized by a considerably enlarged SP and SP:AP amplitude ratio. The corresponding audiogram is fairly symmetrical, with the notable exception that the left ear is 20 dB less sensitive than the right at 250Hz. On the day these tracings were obtained, this patient's symptoms included aural fullness/pressure, tinnitus, and vertigo—all localized to the left side.

Figure 1-6 displays an ECochG intensity series from a normal ear (left tracings), and from an ear with suspected endolymphatic hydrops (right tracings). As HL is reduced in 10-dB steps, both series show the characteristic reduction of AP amplitude and prolongation of N_1 latency. The SP component of the normal tracings decreases to the level of being indistinguishable at 65 dB HL. This reduction in the SP is expected as the system becomes more linear (or less non-linear), at lower HLs. In the hydropic ear, however, the SP is enlarged and appears to persist until the AP is no longer visible.

Another aspect worth noting in Figure 1-6 is that the threshold of N_1 is between 55–45 dB HL in the normal ear, and 65–55 dB HL in the hydropic ear. We have recorded N_1 thresholds as low as 35 dB HL in normal ears, which were elevated in comparison to behavioral thresholds to the same stimulus. Some investigators (e.g., Gibson et al., 1977) have reported good correlation between behavioral and transtympanic electrocochleographic thresholds. Our experience, however, is that Wave V of the ABR persists longer, and is a much better predictor of behavioral threshold in the 2000–4000Hz range than is N_1 of the extratympanically recorded ECochG response. It has also been our experience that high-frequency hearing loss (i.e., in the 2000–4000Hz range) in excess of 60–65 dB HL precludes the recording of reliable and consistent extratympanic ECochG components.

CASE STUDIES

The following section presents clinical case studies from our laboratory wherein ECochG was part of the diagnostic test battery. All recordings were made in the manner previously described in this chapter.

CASE 1

Case 1 was that of a 65-year-old man whose presenting symptoms included bilateral hearing loss, with tinnitus and aural fullness/pressure localized to the left ear. Although he had a history of vertigo, this symptom was not present on the day the ECochG examination was conducted. Electronystagmography (ENG) performed on a prior date revealed left peripheral vestibular hypofunction. His ABR was within normal limits.

This patient's pure-tone audiogram is illustrated in Figure 1-7. The audiogram revealed bilateral hearing loss that was relatively flat up to and including 2000Hz, but dropped off at the higher frequencies and was more pronounced in the left ear. The patient's speech reception thresholds (SRTs) were 25 and 45 dB HL for the right and left ears, respectively. Discrimination maximum for phonetically-balanced (PB) words was 100 percent for the right ear and 84 percent for the left. Tympanograms were normal bilaterally.

ECochG data for this patient are shown in Figure 1-8. The left response was characterized by a considerably enlarged SP, making the left SP:AP amplitude ratio larger than normal. Right ECochG tracings were within normal limits. It is important to note that his hydropic symptoms of tinnitus and aural fullness/pressure were localized to the left ear. These symptoms were objectively supported by ECochG responses.

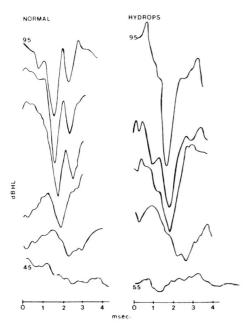

Figure 1-6. ECochG intensity series from a normal subject (left) and from a patient with suspected endolymphatic hydrops (right). Hearing level is reduced in 10-dB steps.

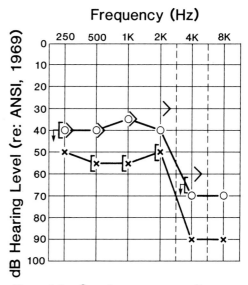

Figure 1-7. Case 1—pure-tone audiogram.

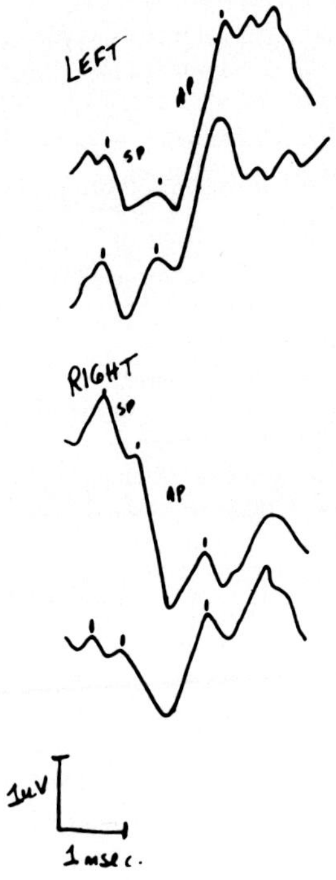

		SP	AP	SP/AP Amplitude Ratio	N$_1$ Latency
LEFT	Duration (msec)	0.70	1.00		
	Amplitude (μV)	0.80	0.30	2.7	1.6 msec
	Duration	0.80	0.90		
	Amplitude	0.80	0.20	4.0	1.7 msec
RIGHT	Duration	0.50	1.00		
	Amplitude	0.85	2.10	0.40	1.6 msec
	Duration	0.40	1.20		
	Amplitude	0.20	0.90	0.22	1.6 msec

Figure 1-8.   Case 1—ECochG data.

CASE 2

Case 2 was that of a 6-year-old child whose symptoms on the day of the ECochG examination included bilateral aural fullness/pressure, bilateral tinnitus, and dysequilibrium. She had spinal meningitis when she was 1 year old, accompanied by a fever of 105°F.

This child's pure-tone audiogram is illustrated in Figure 1-9 and revealed bilateral hearing loss of differing configuration between ears. SRT was 20 and 22 dB HL for left and right ears, respectively, and PB maximum was 96 percent in both ears. Tympanograms were within normal limits bilaterally, as was the ABR.

ECochG data, which is shown in Figure 1-10, revealed a bilateral enlargement of the SP and SP:AP amplitude ratio. There was also a considerable difference, of 0.5 msec, between left and right N_1 latencies. This may be accounted for by the difference in audiometric configuration between ears, and by the fact that this patient's high-frequency sensitivity was better on the left than on the right.

The combination of findings for this patient, and the EcochG responses in particular, suggested the presence of bilateral endolymphatic hydrops. This was also consistent with her symptomatic history.

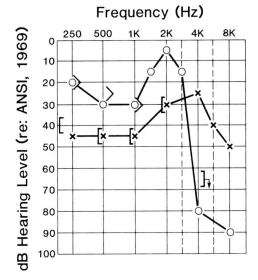

Figure 1-9. Case 2—pure-tone audiogram.

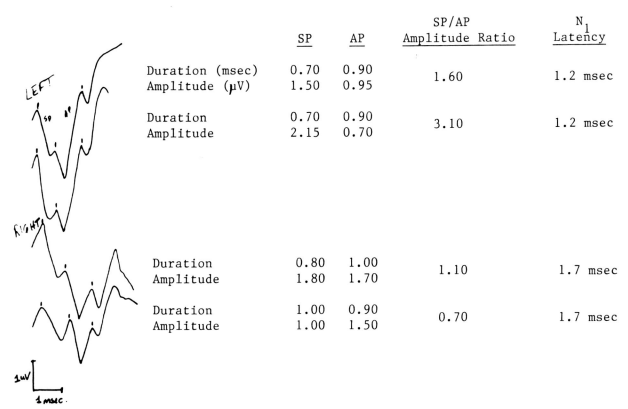

	SP	AP	SP/AP Amplitude Ratio	N_1 Latency
Duration (msec)	0.70	0.90	1.60	1.2 msec
Amplitude (μV)	1.50	0.95		
Duration	0.70	0.90	3.10	1.2 msec
Amplitude	2.15	0.70		
Duration	0.80	1.00	1.10	1.7 msec
Amplitude	1.80	1.70		
Duration	1.00	0.90	0.70	1.7 msec
Amplitude	1.00	1.50		

Figure 1-10. Case 2—ECochG data.

Frequency (Hz)

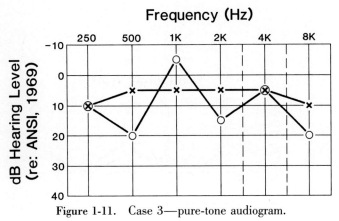

Figure 1-11.   Case 3—pure-tone audiogram.

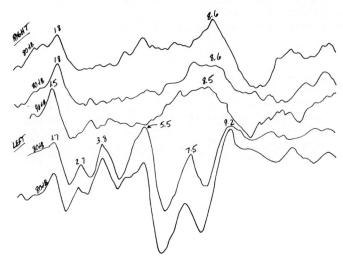

Figure 1-13.   Case 3—auditory brainstem response tracings.

CASE 3

Case 3 was that of a 36-year-old female who had a 3-month history of aural fullness with accompanying tinnitus in her right ear. At the onset of her tinnitus, she stated that she thought "a smoke alarm was going off" before realizing that the sound was coming from her ear.

As can be seen from the audiogram in Figure 1-11, her hearing was virtually normal, bilaterally. SRT was 10 dB HL in the right ear, and 8 dB HL in the left. PB maximum was 92 and 96 percent for the right and left ears, respectively. The Rush Hughes discrimination test was also administered, resulting in a score of 48 percent for the right ear and 72 percent for the left. Tympanograms were normal bilaterally.

Figure 1-12 displays this patient's ECochG tracings. As should now be evident to the reader, these responses were within normal limits bilaterally, save for a slight delay of N_1 latency in the right waveforms. Figure 1-13 displays her

ABRs. The left response was within normal limits, whereas the right response was grossly abnormal. Wave I was well-defined and repeatable, but Wave V was distorted and significantly delayed. The I-V interwave latency was approximately 6.7 msec, which was well beyond our normal limits. Waves II, III, and IV were indiscernible.

Subsequent computerized tomography (CT) examination revealed a mass in the region of the cerebellopontine (CP) angle that eventually proved to be an acoustic neuroma approximately 1 cm² in size.

Case 3 highlights that benefit of combining the results of perhaps several diagnostic tests to produce the most complete and accurate assessment of the patient's status. This is illustrated even more dramatically in Case 4.

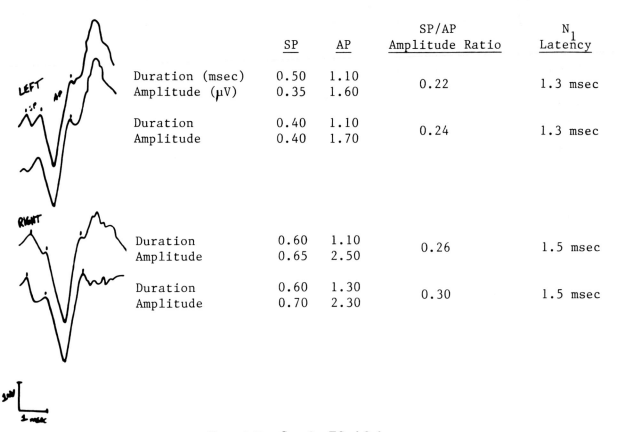

	SP	AP	SP/AP Amplitude Ratio	N_1 Latency
Duration (msec)	0.50	1.10	0.22	1.3 msec
Amplitude (μV)	0.35	1.60		
Duration	0.40	1.10	0.24	1.3 msec
Amplitude	0.40	1.70		
Duration	0.60	1.10	0.26	1.5 msec
Amplitude	0.65	2.50		
Duration	0.60	1.30	0.30	1.5 msec
Amplitude	0.70	2.30		

Figure 1-12.   Case 3—ECochG data.

CASE 4

Case 4 was that of a 60-year-old female who had a 25-year history of symptoms generally associated with endolymphatic hydrops. These included periodic episodes of vertigo, tinnitus, and aural fullness/pressure. The episodes would last approximately 1–2 weeks then disappear, sometimes for as long as 5 years. All symptoms appeared to be localized to the right side. She had been treated medically with a wide variety of drugs, primarily for the relief of her vertigo.

Figure 1-14 illustrates her pure-tone audiogram, which was virtually normal, especially considering her age and symptoms. SRT was 15 dB HL in both ears and PB maximum was 100 percent bilaterally. Once again, there was a noticeable difference in discrimination scores for the Rush Hughes test. The score for the left ear was 76 percent, whereas she was only able to discriminate 56 percent of the words presented to her right ear.

ECochG data from this patient are displayed in Figure 1-15. As can be seen from her tracings, the right response was characterized by an enlarged SP and SP:AP amplitude ratio. The left response was normal.

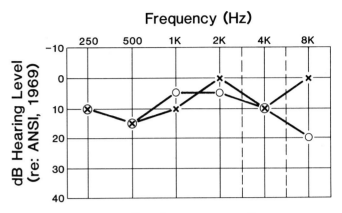

Figure 1-14.   Case 4—pure-tone audiogram.

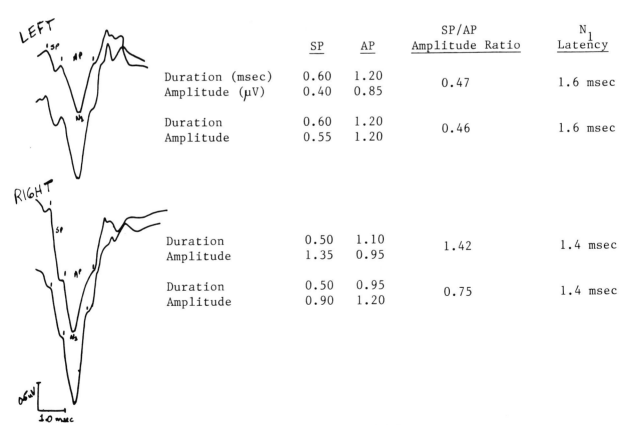

	SP	AP	SP/AP Amplitude Ratio	N_1 Latency
Duration (msec)	0.60	1.20	0.47	1.6 msec
Amplitude (μV)	0.40	0.85		
Duration	0.60	1.20	0.46	1.6 msec
Amplitude	0.55	1.20		
Duration	0.50	1.10	1.42	1.4 msec
Amplitude	1.35	0.95		
Duration	0.50	0.95	0.75	1.4 msec
Amplitude	0.90	1.20		

Figure 1-15.   Case 4—ECochG data.

The sinusoidal harmonic acceleration test (SHAT) was also administered to this patient and the results are shown in Figure 1-16. The reader is referred to an article by Best et al. (1983) for a description of the SHAT and its application in the diagnosis of vestibular dysfunction. The results of the SHAT for this patient revealed that the phase lag between eye and head movement was abnormal at rotational frequencies of 0.005Hz and 0.01Hz (also at 0.16Hz). According to Best et al. (1983), low-frequency phase lag is generally a reflection of peripheral vestibular hypofunction.

Considering that this patient's initial CT scan was normal, the combination of ECochG and SHAT results, in conjunction with her symptomatic history, supports the diagnosis of MD/ELH.

ABR tracings from this patient are displayed in Figure 1-17. The left ABR was within normal limits, whereas the right tracings showed a prolongation of the I-V and I-III interwave latencies. Based on this finding, a CT scan with air contrast was performed, which revealed the presence of a space-occupying lesion in the CP angle. This tumor was later identified during its surgical removal as a meningioma.

Of interest in this particular case, was that the ECochG waveform displayed an enlarged SP:AP amplitude ratio, which suggested the presence of endolymphatic hydrops. This may not have been a "false-positive" finding, however. Schindler (1980), for example, has observed histopathological alterations in the endolymphatic sac of patients with acoustic neuromas.

Once again, the full diagnostic benefit for this patient was realized through the combination of results from several tests. Key amongst them in this case, however, was the ABR.

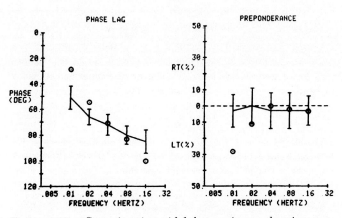

Figure 1-16. Case 4—sinusoidal harmonic acceleration test results.

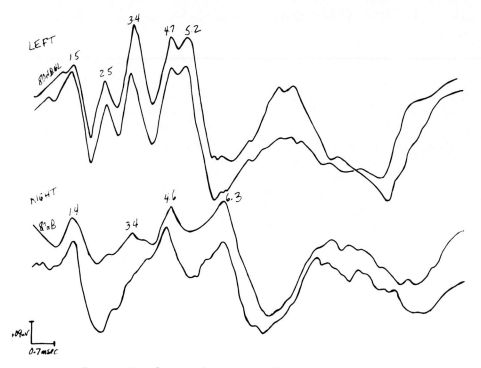

Figure 1-17. Case 4—brainstem auditory response tracings.

ADDITIONAL CONSIDERATIONS

The incidence of abnormal ECochG responses (i.e., enlarged SPs or SP : AP amplitude ratios) in the MD/ELH population has been generally reported to be between 60 and 65 percent (Gibson et al., 1977; Kitahara et al., 1981; Coats 1981; Goin et al., 1982). Examination of our case studies however, reveals that there may be a relationship between ECochG findings and the symptoms of inner ear dysfunction for a given patient. The implication is that the results of an ECochG exam may be influenced by the symptoms, or true inner ear pressure the patient has at the time of testing. These symptoms, in turn, may vary over time due to the pathophysiology of the disease.

We examined this notion by obtaining electrocochleograms from 55 consecutive patients (110 ears) who were referred for testing because of symptoms suggestive of MD/ELH (Ferraro et al., 1985). These symptoms included fluctuating sensorineural hearing loss, vertigo, tinnitus, aural fullness/pressure, and all combinations of these four. Although all patients had a symptomatic history of MD/ELH, several were asymptomatic when ECochG was administered. The results of the ECochG exam were then compared to the symptoms the patients had at the time of testing. This study revealed two important findings regarding the application of ECochG in this population.

The first finding is that ECochG responses were indeed influenced by the symptoms presented at the time of testing. There was a significant difference between ECochG findings when symptoms were absent compared to when one or more of the above symptoms were present.

The second finding is that the strongest "predictor" of an abnormal or positive electrocochleogram was the presence among the symptoms of hearing loss *and* aural fullness/pressure. Given this information, in turn, it was possible to accurately predict the outcome of an ECochG exam 92 percent of the time.

Two important questions arise from the results of the above study. First, if ECochG findings can be predicted based on the patient's symptoms at the time of testing, is there a need for the test at all? Second, if an ECochG exam is scheduled, should it be performed if the patient is asymptomatic?

Our experience suggests that the answer to both of these questions may be yes, with certain qualifications. Regarding the first question, ECochG seems to provide an objective indication of what may be a very subjective symptom(s) (e.g., aural fullness or pressure). This information, in turn, may be useful in substantiating a diagnosis, justifying treatment regimens, and monitoring the effects of treatment. It would be interesting, in fact, to conduct similar studies with other tests such as electronystagmography, auditory dehydration tests, and sinusoidal harmonic acceleration, which have also been used to diagnose MD/ELH.

With respect to the second question, our data and experience suggest that if an exam is performed when the patient is asymptomatic or between attacks, the exam should be repeated for comparative purposes when the patient is experiencing symptoms, especially hearing loss and aural fullness/pressure. This may, in fact, be the most effective way to apply ECochG in the MD/ELH population. The feasibility of this, however, is questionable due to the pathophysiology and "capricious" nature of the disease(s), as well as the operating times and scheduling limitations of most clinics. The decision to administer an exam, therefore, may depend on a variety of both subjective and objective factors. Based on our data, however, the value of an ECochG exam performed on an asymptomatic patient is questionable, unless the exam is repeated when the patient has symptoms. On the other hand, if the initial exam is performed when the patient is symptomatic, the diagnostic relevance of repeat exams decreases.

Another factor to consider regarding the clinical application of ECochG is that in comparison to the ABR, for example, it is generally more difficult and time-consuming to obtain repeatable, well-defined, and clinically useful ECochG tracings. This is due in part to procedural factors. For example, the expanded band-pass of the pre-amplifier filter will allow more "noise" into the system. In addition, electrode contact and stability, as well as ear canal configuration, contribute to response variability across and within subjects. Waveform variability may also be due to factors inherent to the responses being recorded. The SP evoked by click stimuli, for example, is often inconsistent and difficult to define even under ideal recording conditions.

Despite the above limitations, we have found electrocochleography to be a useful and important component of our auditory evoked response test battery. This is especially true in the objective identification, assessment, and monitoring of Meniere's disease and endolymphatic hydrops. Continued advancements in our understanding of the electrophysiological events associated with hearing, as well as in the technological aspects of recording these events, will most certainly facilitate and extend the clinical application of ECochG. In essence, we have yet to derive the full benefit of a noninvasive, painless tool that provides a "window" through which we can study the physiology and pathophysiology of the human ear.

ACKNOWLEDGMENT

The author would like to extend his appreciation to Nancy Martin for her clerical assistance in the preparation of this manuscript.

REFERENCES

Andreev, AM, & Aropova, AA, Gersuni, SV (1939). On electrical potentials in the human cochlea. *J Physiol, USSR, 26*, 205–212

Best, LG, Ferraro, JA, Arenberg, IK (1983). The clinical value of computerized sinusoidal harmonic acceleration testing in patients with endolymphatic hydrops. *Otolaryngol Clin North Am, 16*, 83–93

Coats, AC, Dickey, JR (1970). Non-surgical recording of human auditory-nerve action potentials and cochlear microphonics. *Ann Otol Rhinol Laryngol, 29*, 844–851

Coats, AC (1974). On electrocochleographic electrode design. *J Acoust Soc Am, 56*, 708–711

Coats, AC (1981). Meniere's disease and the summating potential: II. Vestibular test results. *Arch Otolaryngol, 107*, 263–270

Cullen, JK, & Ellis, MS, Berlin, CI, Lousteau, RJ (1972). Human nerve action potential recordings from the tympanic membrane without anesthesia. *Acta Otolaryngol, 74*, 15–22

Cullen, JL, Berlin, CI, Gondra, MI, Adams, ML (1976). Electrocochleography in children: A retrospective study. *Arch Otolaryngol, 102*, 482

FERRARO

Dallos, P, Schoeny, ZG, Cheatham, MA (1972). Cochlear summating potentials: Descriptive aspects. *Acta Otolaryngol, 301 (Suppl.)*, 1–46

Dallos, P (1973). *The auditory periphery: Biophysics and physiology.* New York: Academic Press

Davis, H, Fernandez, C, McAuliffe, DR (1950). The excitatory process in the cochlea. *Proc Natl Acad Sci, 36*, 580–587

Durrant, JD, Dallos, P (1972). Influence of direct-current polarization of the cochlear partition on the summating potential. *J Acoust Soc Am, 52*, 542–552

Durrant, JD, Gans, D (1977). Biasing of the summating potentials. *Acta Otolaryngol, 80*, 13–18

Elberling, C, Salomon, G (1973). Cochlear microphonic recorded from the ear canal in man. *Acta Otolaryngol, 75*, 489–495

Ferraro JA, Best, LG, Arenberg, IK (1983). The use of electrocochleography in the diagnosis, assessment and monitoring of endolymphatic hydrops. *Otolaryngol Clin North Am, 16*, 69–82

Ferraro JA, Arenberg IK, Hassanein RS (1985). Electrocochleography and symptoms of inner ear dysfunction. *Arch Otolaryngol, 111*, 71–74

Ferraro JA, Ruth, RA (1985). Clinical electrocochleography. *Hearing Journal, 38*, 51–55

Ferraro, JA, Murphy, GB, Ruth, RA (1986). A comparative study of primary electrodes used in extratympanic electrocochleography. In JA Ferraro (Ed.), *Electrocochleography, seminars in hearing.* New York: Thieme-Stratton

Fromm, B, Bylen, CO, Zotterman, Y (1935). Studies in the mechanisms of Wever and Bray effect. *Acta Otolaryngol, 22*, 477–483

Gerhardt, HJ, Wagner, H, Werbs, M (1985). Electrocochleography (ECochG) and brain stem evoked response recordings (BSER) in the diagnosis of acoustic neuromas. *Acta Otolaryngol, 99*, 384–386

Gibbin, KP, Mason, ST, Majumdar, B (1983). Investigation of Meniere's disorder by extratympanic electrocochleography. *Adv Otorhinolaryngol, 31*, 198–207

Gibson, WPR, Beagley, MA (1976). Transtympanic electrocochleography in the investigation of retrocochlear disorders. *Revue Laryngol, 97 (Suppl.)*, 507–516

Gibson, WPR, Moffat, DA, Ramsden, RT (1977). Clinical electrocochleography in the diagnosis and management of Meniere's disorder. *Audiology, 16*, 389–401

Gibson, WPR (1978). *Essentials of electric response audiometry.* New York: Churchill and Livingstone

Goin, DW, Staller, SJ, Asher, DL, Mischke, RE (1982). Summating potential in Meniere's disease. *Laryngoscope, 92*, 1383–1389

Jewett, DL, Williston, JS (1971). Auditory evoked far fields averaged from the scalp of humans. *Brain, 94*, 681–696

Kiang, NS (1965). Discharge patterns of single nerve fibers in the cat's auditory nerve. Research Monograph 35, Cambridge, MA: MIT Press

Kitahara, M, Takeda, T, Yazama, T (1981). Electrocochleography in the diagnosis of Meniere's disease. In KH Volsten (Ed.), *Meniere's disease, pathogenesis, diagnosis and treatment.* New York: Thieme-Stratton

Kumagami, H, Nishida, H, Masaaki, B (1982). Electrocochleographic study of Meniere's disease. *Arch Otolaryngol, 108*, 284–288

Lempert, J, Wever, EG, Lawrence, M (1947). The cochleogram and its clinical applications: A preliminary report. *Arch Otolaryngol, 45*, 61–67

Lempert, J, Meltzer, PE, Wever, EG, Lawrence, M (1950). The cochleogram and its clinical applications: Concluding observations. *Arch Otolaryngol, 51*, 307–311

Moriuchi, H, Kumagami, H (1979). Changes of AP, SP and CM in experimental endolymphatic hydrops. *Audiology, 22*, 258–260

Morrison, AW, Moffat, DA, O'Connor, AF (1980). Clinical usefulness of electrocochleography in Meniere's disease: An analysis of dehydrating agents. *Otolaryngol Clin North Am, 11*, 703–721

Perlman, MB, Case, TJ (1941). Electrical phenomena of the cochlea in man. *Arch Otolaryngol, 34*, 710–718

Portmann, M, Aran, JM (1972). Relations entre pattern electrocochleographique et pathologie retrolabyrintique. *Acta Otolaryngol, 73*, 190–196

Ronis, BJ (1966). Cochlear potentials in otosclerosis. *Laryngoscope, 76*, 212–231

Ruben, RJ, Sekula, J, Bordley, JE (1960). Human cochlear responses to sound stimuli. *Ann Otorhinolaryngol, 69*, 459–476

Schindler, RA (1980). The ultrastructure of the endolymphatic cac in man. *Laryngoscope, 90 (Suppl. 21)*, 1–79

Schmidt, PH, Eggermont, JT, Odenthal, DW (1974). Study of Meniere's disease by electrocochleography. *Acta Otolaryngol, 316 (Suppl.)*, 75–84

Sohmer, H, Feinmesser, M (1967). Cochlear action potentials recorded from the external ear in man. *Ann Otolaryngol, 76*, 427–435

Tasaki, I, Davis, H, Eldredge, DH (1954). Exploration of cochlear potentials in guinea pig with a micro-electrode. *J Acoust Soc Am, 26*, 765–773

von Bekesy, G (1950). DC potentials and energy balance of the cochlear partition. *J Acoust Soc Am, 22*, 576–582

Wever, EG, Bray, C (1930). Action currents in the auditory nerve in response to acoustic stimulation. *Proc Natl Acad Sci, 16*, 344–350

Whitfield, IC, Ross, HF (1965). Cochlear microphonic and summating potentials and the outputs of individual hair cell generators. *J Acoust Soc Am, 38*, 126–131

Yanz, JL, Dodds, H (1985). An ear-canal electrode for the measurement of the human auditory brain stem response. *Ear Hear, 6*, 98–104

Yoshie, N, Ohashi, T, Suzuki, T (1967). Non-surgical recording of auditory nerve action potentials in man. *Laryngoscope, 77*, 76–81

Jeffrey H. Owen

2

Clinical Audiologic Applications
of Acoustically Elicited Evoked Responses

Behavioral audiometric procedures have traditionally been the method of choice to determine a patient's hearing status. In the difficult-to-test patient, however, alternative techniques may be necessary because behavioral methods are not clinically or economically feasible. One alternative technique is evoked potential (EP) testing. The objective is to generate a physiologically based audiogram that can be used for habilititation or rehabilitation. Because the patient is difficult-to-test, it is typically necessary to use sedation. Consequently, the EP procedure must not be too long, nor should the sedation adversely influence test results.

The purpose of this chapter is to provide a brief review of the potentials elicited by acoustical signals, the methods used to elicit them, and the strengths and weaknesses of these potentials as they pertain to the difficult-to-test patient. Normative and clinical data elicited by these and other audiological procedures will be presented.

CLASSIFICATION OF POTENTIALS

Acoustically elicited potentials are typically classified according to their time of occurrence (e.g., early, middle, late) or their anatomical site(s) of origin (e.g., cochlear, brainstem, cortical). Table 2-1 depicts a version of a classification scheme reported in Owen and Davis, 1985.

COCHLEAR RESPONSES

The cochlear responses consist of the cochlear microphonic, summating potential, and the action potential of cranial nerve (CN)VIII. These potentials have been thoroughly reviewed

and their clinical utility discussed in the chapter on electrocochleography (Chapter 1) by Dr. John Ferraro, in this atlas. The reader is referred to that chapter for additional information on these responses.

EARLY RESPONSES

Early responses occur within 2–15 msec following stimulus presentation and originate in the auditory nerve and brainstem structures. These responses are all-or-none axonal potentials and represent the non-sequential activation of parallel circuitry within the auditory system. Collectively, these responses are known as the brainstem auditory evoked response (BAER). The best-known BAER is the Jewett series (Jewett and Williston, 1971), which is elicited by a transient signal known as a click.

The BAER demonstrates several audiological advantages that make it useful for evaluating the difficult-to-test patient. First, subject state and sedation do not influence the response. Rather, sleep, either natural or induced, actually improves the

Table 2-1 Classification of Auditory Evoked Responses

Response	Latency Range	Origin
Cochlear	0–4 msec	Cochlea
Early	2–15 msec	CN VIII and brainstem
Middle	15–50 msec	Brainstem, midbrain, auditory cortex
Late	50–300 msec	Primary and secondary auditory cortex

Clinical Atlas of Auditory Evoked Potentials
ISBN 0-8089-1896-6

detection of the response at very low sensation levels (SLs). This results in closer agreement between the behavioral and physiological thresholds to the same stimulus. Second, when using a click, valuable information regarding the neurological status of brainstem auditory structures is also obtained.

The major disadvantage of the BAER is that the acoustically transduced click is broadband in its frequency spectrum. Consequently, click-elicited BAERs provide minimal information regarding auditory sensitivity at specific test frequencies, especially in the low and mid-frequencies. This disadvantage has been virtually eliminated by utilizing the BAER procedure known as the slow-negative-10 (SN10) response (Davis and Hirsh, 1979).

The SN10 response is a scalp-negative potential that can be elicited using tone burst stimuli centered at specific frequencies. This response now appears to be the method of choice for generating a physiologically based audiogram. Normative data are presented in Figures 2-1 through 2-5. These data were elicited from a normal hearing, awake adult using clicks and tone bursts centered at 500, 1000, 2000, and 4000Hz. Reliable and morphologically identifiable responses were obtained at intensity levels as low as 25 dB SL (re: the subject's behavioral threshold to the test stimuli) for all 5 stimuli. Data can typically be obtained at even lower SLs when the subject has been sedated.

It should be noted that when using SN10/BAER procedures clinically, we typically do not present stimuli at intensity levels less than 25 dB nHL (re: normal hearing level). This is based upon the assumption that hearing sensitivity better than 25 dB nHL typically does not produce significant reductions in speech and/or language development. Presenting stimuli at lower inten-

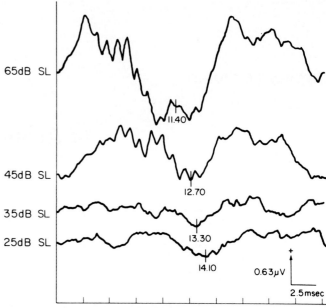

Figure 2-2. Normative SN10 data elicited by a 500Hz tone burst presented at various intensity levels.

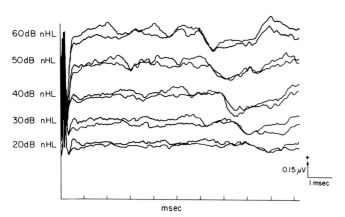

Figure 2-1. Click elicited BAER data obtained from a normal hearing adult at various intensity levels.

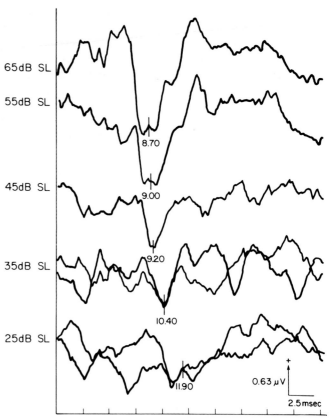

Figure 2-3. Normative data elicited by a 1000Hz tone burst presented at various intensity levels.

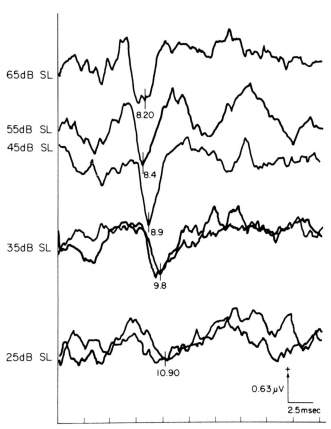

Figure 2-4. Normative data elicited by a 2000Hz tone burst presented at various intensity levels.

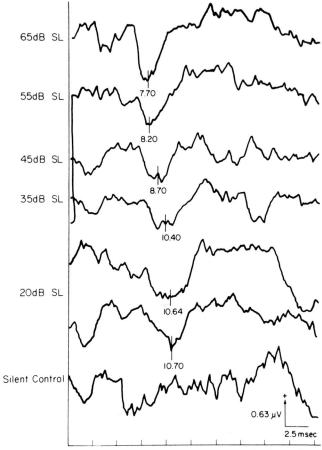

Figure 2-5. Normative data elicited by a 4000Hz tone burst presented at various intensity levels.

sity levels will, however, increase the duration of the examination, when time is already limited, especially when sedation is used. Figure 2-6 depicts the procedural guide we use to determine response threshold. Inspection of this table reveals that the presence of a response is determined primarily by its morphology and reliability. By using this guide, we have found that reliable and valid estimations of behavioral thresholds are obtained in the shortest amount of time.

Duration of the test session is a critical component when evaluating the difficult-to-test patient, particularly under sedation. When using chloral hydrate, the duration of sedation time is typically 1 hour. Our protocol involves first using click stimuli to elicit the BAER. This will provide an estimate of high-frequency hearing and determine the neurological status of the patient's auditory system. If necessary, stimuli are then presented in the following order: 1000Hz, 500Hz, 2000Hz, and 4000Hz. Thresholds are obtained in each ear, before changing to a different stimulus frequency.

Tables 2-2 and 2-3 list mean normative latency values and standard deviations of click-elicited BAER and SN10 data obtained at various intensity levels and frequencies. Data were elicited from audiologically and neurologically normal adults and infants who were sedated or sleeping naturally. Data listed in these tables indicate that as intensity level and/or frequency are decreased, latency of the response increases. Additionally,

Table 2-2 Tone Burst-Elicited Infant and Adult Normative Data

	Mean		Standard Deviation	
Stimulus	Infant	Adult	Infant	Adult
500Hz				
60 dB	11.85	12.06	0.55	0.20
40 dB	13.68	14.00	0.83	0.20
20 dB	15.38	20.00	0.80	0.20
1000Hz				
60 dB	10.36	10.00	0.39	0.40
40 dB	11.38	12.00	0.76	0.30
20 dB	14.01	14.03	0.87	0.35
2000Hz				
60 dB	9.58	9.70	0.32	0.20
40 dB	10.32	10.50	0.30	0.30
20 dB	11.75	12.00	0.52	0.50
4000Hz				
60 dB	9.02	8.80	0.23	0.20
40 dB	9.90	10.00	0.26	0.23
20 dB	11.23	11.50	0.69	0.51

All dB values are re: normal hearing adult thresholds.

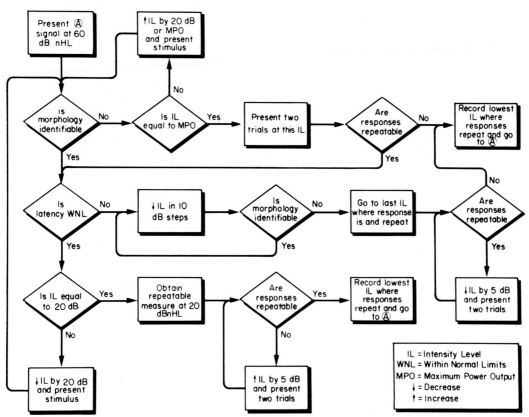

Figure 2-6. Decision-making flow chart used to determine the presence of a response during audiological testing.

Table 2-3 Click-elicited Infant and Adult Normative Data

Stimulus	Mean Infant	Mean Adult	Standard Deviation Infant	Standard Deviation Adult
65 dB				
Wave I	1.76	1.64	0.20	0.10
Wave III	4.35	3.79	0.12	0.13
Wave V	6.39	5.73	0.18	0.17
45 dB				
Wave I	2.50	2.16	0.32	0.18
Wave III	—	4.40	—	0.23
Wave V	7.04	6.38	0.22	0.21
25 dB				
Wave I	—	—	—	—
Wave III	—	—	—	—
Wave V	7.39	6.63	0.25	0.23

All dB values are re: normal hearing adult thresholds.

as the patient's age increases, up to approximately 2–3 years of age, the latency of the response continues to decrease.

Since sedation is usually required to evaluate the difficult-to-test patient, the examiner must be aware of its effects on test results. When using chloral hydrate or secobarbital, the BAER is not deleteriously influenced. Various dosage schedules for chloral hydrate are available. Davis (Owen and Davis, 1985) has presented a useful schedule for administering secobarbital.

MIDDLE–LATE RESPONSES

The middle and late responses are acoustically elicited electrical events that originate within higher neural structures than does the BAER. Both responses probably represent dendritic activity. Following stimulus presentation, the middle response occurs within 15–40 msec and the late response within 50–300 msec (Davis and Owen, 1985).

There are several audiological advantages to using these responses. First, both responses can be elicited by clicks and tone bursts. Second, both responses can be elicited by low-frequency tone bursts (i.e., 250 Hz). This is an obvious advantage when developing a physiologically based audiogram. Third, response threshold is usually very close to the patient's behavioral threshold to the same stimulus. It is not unusual that these 2 thresholds are within 5–10 dB of each other.

There are two significant audiological disadvantages to the middle and late responses. First, subject state influences the response. Because the response originates in high brainstem and cortical structures, subject state and state-altering drugs influence response morphology, latency, and reliability (see Case 1). Consequently, the response elicited from an awake patient will be significantly different when elicited from the same individual under sedation. This is complicated even more because subject state fluctuates during sleep or sedation, which reduces within-test-session reliability.

The second disadvantage of these responses is that they can be contaminated by muscle artifact. Muscle artifact is a factor because its frequency characteristics and those of the bandpass filter used during the test are very similar. Changing bandpass filter characteristics will reduce the noise, but it will also change the response.

While these responses should be considered for use with the cooperative, awake patient, this is not the typical testing situation with the difficult-to-test patient. In most cases, if the patient is quiet and cooperative, traditional behavioral methods could be and should be used. In the less than ideal situation, BAER methods should be considered.

ACQUISITION PARAMETERS

The parameters used to elicit/record the various auditory evoked potentials are listed in Table 2-4. Because each response has its own characteristics, the parameters used to ac-

Table 2-4 Acquisition Parameters

Parameter	Click-BAER	Response SN10	Middle	Late
Stimulus	click	tone burst	clicks or tone bursts	
Frequency	N/A	500, 1k, 2k	500, 1000, 2000, 4000Hz	
Rise	instantaneous	2 cycles	instanteous	5 msec
Plateau	100 μsec	1 cycle	100 μsec	22 msec
Decay	instantaneous	2 cycles	instanteous	5 msec
Rate	11.1/sec	32.3/sec	39.1/sec	0.5/sec
LLF	150Hz	50Hz	5Hz	1Hz
HLF	3000Hz	1700Hz	100Hz	30Hz
Window	10 msec adults 15 msec infants	25 msec	50 msec	750 msec
Polarity	rarefaction	alternating	single or alternating	
Sample	2000	2000	1500	32

quire the response differ. In general, as the origin of the response becomes more central, the bandpass filter emphasizes the lower frequencies, presentation rate decreases, and the analysis window increases. Except for cochlear potentials, the same electrode montage can generally be used for the BAER, middle, and late responses (Owen, 1982).

TESTING PROTOCOL

As has traditionally been the case in medicine, the presence or absence of a pathology, audiologic or otherwise, is based upon the results of a number of diagnostic tests. In the audiology clinic, this necessitates the administration of procedures sensitive to middle-ear, cochlear, and retrocochlear pathologies. Prior to administering evoked potentials for audiologic purposes, the audiologist must first determine the functional and neurological status of the auditory system. This is best accomplished by first assessing the middle ear and proceeding in a central direction. Our protocol assesses the middle ear using immittance and acoustic reflex methods.

When administering immittance procedures to infants, care must be taken to avoid spurious results due to increased mobility or collapsing of the ear canals. Additionally, ipsilateral acoustic reflexes can be erroneous if the probe and reflex-eliciting tones are not multiplexed.

Following middle-ear assessment, the neurologic status of the auditory system must be determined. This is most easily accomplished using click elicited BAERs. Based upon these data, it is possible to ascertain the operating characteristics of the auditory system to repetitive stimuli, as well as to rule out a number of neurologic pathologies. While the majority of these pathologies are typically not present in the difficult-to-test patient, this information is helpful when interpreting data for audiologic purposes. For example, we have found that the neurological activity elicited by repetitive stimuli is often asynchronous in post-meningitic patients. This will result in a degradation of the response and an overestimation of the physiological threshold to the test stimulus.

An additional benefit of elicitng the BAER to click stimuli is that an estimate of auditory sensitivity in the 2000–4000 Hz range is obtained. This is beneficial because it provides the examiner with information regarding the frequency area demonstrating the highest incidence of hearing loss. Such indirect information can be useful for planning the test session, especially when sedation is used. After determining thresholds for click stimuli, we elicit the SN10 response to stimuli presented in the following order: 1000, 500, 2000, and 4000Hz. This order of presentation quickly provides us with information at those frequencies necessary for speech and language development. We also obtain thresholds in each ear before changing frequency. This provides us with information regarding auditory status in each ear, which can be helpful in the event the patient awakens from sedation.

Evaluating the auditory sensitivity of patients using evoked potential procedures is demanding and requires a very systematic approach. A protocol for eliciting and analyzing data is presented in Figure 2-6. Without some type of systematic approach to this procedure, it is very easy to end up with unreliable and invalid test results.

When reporting results, the intensity level of the test signal must be normalized in reference to a standard. We reference all of our data to normal hearing for the same eliciting stimulus. Normalizing the intensity level of the eliciting signal reduces the inherent difference between thresholds to short- and long-duration signals (i.e., tone bursts vs pure tones). As with all applications of evoked potentials, each laboratory must develop its own normative data. This is especially true when short-duration acoustical signals are used to elicit the response. During the interim, published norms may be used. For neurological purposes, statistical ranges of "normality" are used to interpret test results. While we determine similar ranges, interpretation for audiologic purposes is based primarily on the presence/absence of a response.

Another criterion we have found useful in determining the presence or absence of a response at threshold is its amplitude. A response is considered to be present if its amplitude is two-times greater than data collected during a silent control period. By using reliability, latency, and amplitude criteria, it is possible to obtain click and SN10 thresholds consistently within 15 dB of the patient's behavioral threshold to the test stimulus.

Habilitation/Rehabilitation

Our purpose in administering tone burst procedures is to generate a physiologically based audiogram that can be used for habilitative or rehabilitative purposes. A question that often arises regards the discrepancy between behavioral and physiological thresholds, especially as it pertains to fitting a hearing aid or making other recommendations. We have found that our methods provide a very close approximation to the patient's behavioral threshold. Furthermore, commercially available hearing aids demonstrated adequate flexibility to offset any discrepancy between physiological and behavioral thresholds. We have yet to change a recommendation based upon evoked potential data.

After a patient is seen an audiogram is generated, a hearing aid is recommended based upon *all* available test results. Prior to the actual fitting of the aid, we will usually retest the patient at one or more frequencies in order to determine inter-test-session reliability. Final hearing aid recommendation is withheld until otological clearance is obtained and inter-test-session reliability is determined.

CLINICAL DATA

CASE 1

History

This 23-month-old female was diagnosed as having an intraventricular cyst of the fourth ventricle (Dandy-Walker syndrome). In addition, the patient presented a history of recurrent middle-ear infections and delayed speech/language and motor skills.

Test Procedures

Testing consisted of immittance and brainstem audiometry. Clicks and tone bursts centered at 500 and 1000Hz were used to elicit the BAER. The patient was sedated with chloral hydrate throughout the test session.

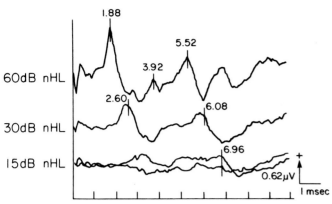

Figure 2-7. Click elicited BAER data obtained from the right ear of the patient described in Case 1.

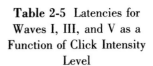

Table 2-5 Latencies for Waves I, III, and V as a Function of Click Intensity Level

		Right	Left
Wave I	60 dB nHL	1.88	1.68
	30 dB nHL	2.60	2.52
	15 dB nHL	3.28	3.48
Wave III	60 dB nHL	3.92	3.76
	30 dB nHL	4.68	4.44
	15 dB nHL	5.40	5.38
Wave V	60 dB nHL	5.52	5.32
	30 dB nHL	6.08	6.12
	15 dB nHL	6.96	6.76

Test Results

Immittance results revealed Type A tympanograms (Feldman & Wilbur, 1976), bilaterally. Acoustic reflex thresholds were within normal limits at 500, 1000, 2000, and 4000Hz, bilaterally.

Click-elicited BAERs were reliabily obtained at 60, 30, and 15 dB nHL, bilaterally (Figs. 2-7 and 2-8). Absolute latencies for the click-BAERs are shown in Table 2-5. Tone-burst elicited BAERs were elicited during the same test session. Actual SN10 data elicited by 500Hz and 1000Hz stimuli are shown in Figures 2-9 and 2-10, respectively. Because results from each ear were nearly identical, only right ear data are shown. Absolute latencies, in msec, of these data are shown in Table 2-6.

Behavioral testing, using operant techniques, was completed by the time this patient was 3 years of age. The behavioral audiometric thresholds shown in Table 2-7 were obtained. Results from both BAER and behavioral techniques were consistent with normal hearing, bilaterally. Readministration of BAER techniques, following the last behavioral test (Fig. 2-11) confirmed initial evoked potential results. It should be noted that evoked potential tests were completed more than 1 year prior to behavioral testing.

During the initial testing of this patient, attempts were made to he elicit the late response using long-duration (22 msec), 1000Hz tone bursts. Figure 2-12 depicts 2 trials of data elicited from the right ear. These data were obviously not reliable and provided no additional information regarding auditory sensitivity.

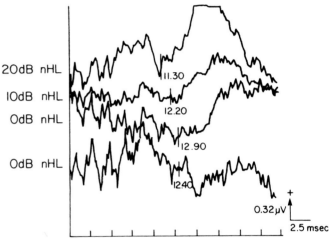

Figure 2-9. SN10 data obtained from the right ear of the patient described in Case 1, using a 500Hz tone burst presented at various SLs.

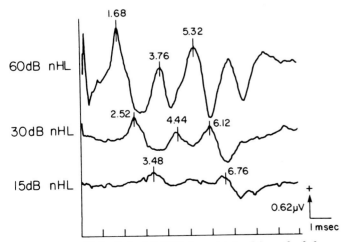

Figure 2-8. Click elicited BAER data obtained from the left ear of the patient described in Case 1.

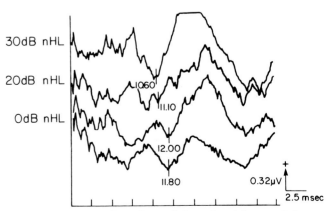

Figure 2-10. SN10 data obtained from the right ear of the patient described in Case 1, using a 1000Hz tone burst presented at various intensity levels.

Table 2-6 Latency of SN10 Response as a Function of Frequency and Intensity Level		Right	Left
500Hz	40 dB nHL	11.30	11.60
	30 dB nHL	12.20	12.50
	20 dB nHL	12.90	13.00
1000Hz	40 dB nHL	10.60	10.80
	30 dB nHL	11.10	11.30
	20 dB nHL	11.80	12.10

Table 2-7 Behavioral Thresholds for Case #1	500Hz	1000Hz	2000Hz	4000Hz
Right	10 dB	5 dB	DNT*	10 dB
Left	10 dB	0 dB	DNT*	10 dB

* DNT = Did not test

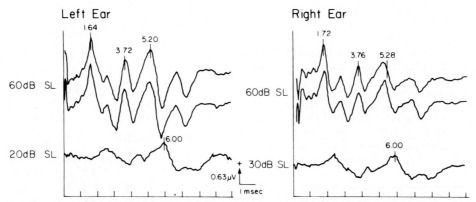

Figure 2-11. Click elicited BAERs obtained from the patient described in Case 1 approximately 13 months following initial testing.

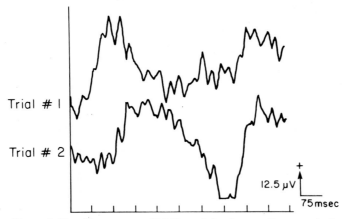

Figure 2-12. Test-retest reliability of the late auditory evoked response elicited from the patient described in Case 1, using a 1000 Hz tone burst.

CASE 2

History

This 2-day-old infant was evaluated because of a reported familial history of hearing loss. The infant was full-term (gestational age of 38 weeks), with no reported complications at birth. Because of this history and the infant's response only to high-intensity stimuli, presented in sound-field, assessment of each ear was requested.

Test Procedures

Because of the high incidence of invalid results in infants, immittance and acoustic reflex tests were not administered. BAERs were elicited using clicks and tone bursts centered at 500, 1000, and 2000Hz. Data were elicited at 60, 40 and 20 dB nHL, and during a silent control.

Test Results

Absolute latencies of click elicited data are shown in Table 2-8.

Data elicited by tonal stimuli presented at 500, 1000, and 2000Hz, using SN10 techniques, are depicted in Figures 2-13 through 2-18. Absolute latencies of these responses were determined, as shown in Table 2-9.

Note that silent control periods, which are very helpful in determining the presence of a response at low SLs, are also depicted. A silent control run consists of presenting stimuli at maximum attenuation, but with all other eliciting and recording parameters held constant. A response is considered to be present when its amplitude is twice that of data obtained during a silent control. The data elicited from this infant were interpreted as being within normal limits and consistent with normal auditory function.

Table 2-8 Click
Latencies as a Function of
Intensity

		Right	Left
Wave I	60 dB	1.96	1.96
	40 dB	2.80	2.72
	20 dB	3.56	3.58
Wave III	60 dB	4.52	4.52
	40 dB	5.20	5.40
	20 dB	6.26	6.44
Wave V	60 dB	6.56	6.52
	40 dB	7.28	7.12
	20 dB	8.04	8.16

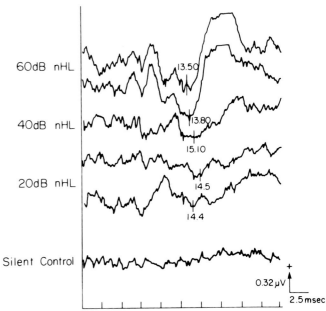

Figure 2-14. SN10 data obtained from the left ear of the patient described in Case 2, using a 500Hz tone burst presented at various intensity levels.

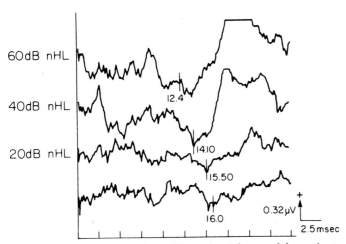

Figure 2-13. SN10 data elicited from the right ear of the patient described in Case 2, using a 500 Hz tone burst presented at various intensity levels.

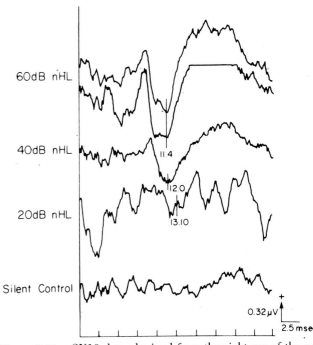

Figure 2-15. SN10 data obtained from the right ear of the patient described in Case 2, using a 1000Hz tone burst presented at various intensity levels.

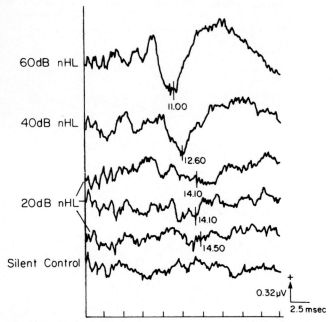

Figure 2-16. SN10 data obtained from the left ear of the patient described in Case 2, using a 1000Hz tone burst presented at various intensity levels.

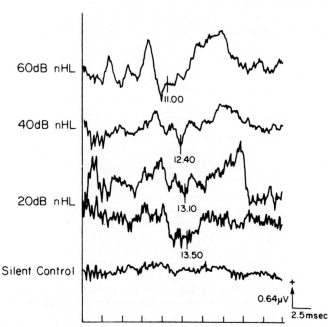

Figure 2-18. SN10 data obtained from the left ear of the patient described in Case 2, using a 2000Hz tone burst presented at various intensity levels.

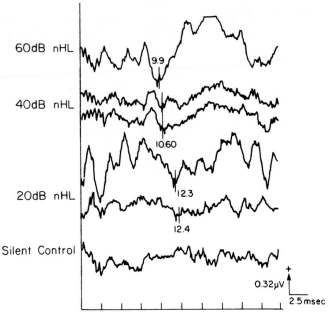

Figure 2-17. SN10 data obtained from the right ear of the patient described in Case 2, using a 2000Hz tone burst presented at various intensity levels.

Table 2-9 SN10
Latencies as a Function of
Frequency and Intensity

		Right	Left
500Hz	60 dB	12.40	13.50
	40 dB	14.10	13.80
	20 dB	15.50	14.50
1000Hz	60 dB	11.40	11.10
	40 dB	12.00	12.60
	20 dB	13.10	14.10
2000Hz	60 dB	9.90	11.00
	40 dB	10.60	12.40
	20 dB	12.40	13.10

CASE 3

History

Case 3 was a 20-month-old with a reported history of inconsistent response to sound. The parents reported that the pregnancy was full-term and the delivery unremarkable. Initially, the infant's responses to sounds were grossly normal, but became inconsistent at approximately 15 months of age. There was no reported history of medical or familial problems pertinent to hearing.

Test Procedures

Testing consisted of administering immittance and acoustic reflex audiometry, and click elicited BAER procedures, bilaterally.

Test Results

Type B tympanograms with an absence of acoustic reflexes at the maximum presentation level of the bridge were obtained, bilaterally. Click elicited data for the right and left ear are depicted in Figures 2-19 through 2-23. Absolute latency values are shown in Table 2-10. Interpretation of test results strongly suggested the presence of a middle-ear pathology. While otoscopic screening of the ear canals ruled out occlusion due to wax, etc., an otological evaluation was requested.

Results from the otological evaluation revealed the presence of serous otitis media, bilaterally. Following otologic treatment, evoked potential procedures were readministered.

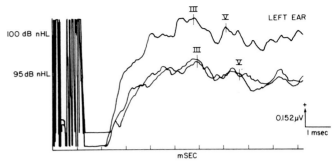

Figure 2-21. Click elicited BAER obtained from the left ear of the patient described in Case 3 during initial test session.

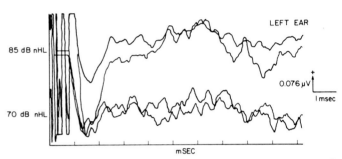

Figure 2-22. Click elicited BAER obtained from the left ear of the patient described in Case 3 during initial test session.

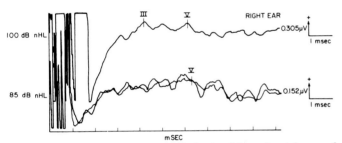

Figure 2-19. Click elicited BAER obtained from the right ear of the patient described in Case 3 during initial test session.

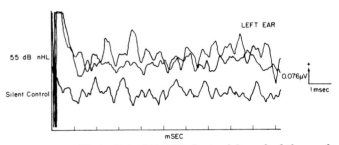

Figure 2-23. Click elicited BAER obtained from the left ear of the patient described in Case 3 during initial test session.

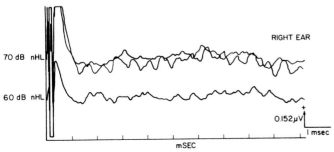

Figure 2-20. Click elicited BAER obtained from the right ear of the patient described in Case 3 during initial test session.

Table 2-10 Click Responses for Case 3		
	Right	Left
Wave I	no reliable Wave I at any intensity level	
Wave III	100 dB 4.20	4.04
Wave V	100 dB 6.14	6.76
	85 dB 6.30 (?)	7.64 at 95 dB
	no reliable Wave V below 85 dB	

Test Results (Session 2)

Type C (−120 mm H₂O) tympanograms with acoustic reflexes within normal limits were obtained, bilaterally. Click elicited BAERs (Figs. 2-24 through 2-27) demonstrated the latencies shown in Table 2-11. Click-elicited data were consistent with grossly normal hearing, bilaterally. Response latencies of click data were considered to be slightly delayed, which was attributed to residual effects of the middle-ear problem. At approximately 26 months of age, behavioral procedures were initiated, and these were completed within 3 months. Behavioral and BAER thresholds were within 5 dB.

This case demonstrates that evoked potential procedures provide the examiner with information regarding the functional status of each ear at an earlier age than is possible using behavioral audiometric techniques. In addition to detecting the presence of a hearing loss, it was possible to ascertain that the loss was conductive in origin. This alerts the parents to the likelihood of continued middle-ear problems with associated reductions in hearing.

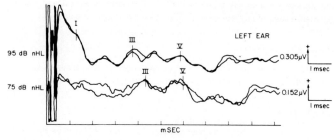

Figure 2-26. Click elicited BAER data obtained from the left ear of the patient described in Case 3 during session 2.

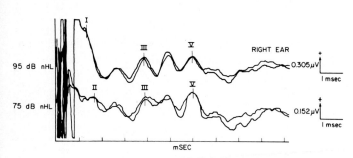

Figure 2-24. Click elicited BAER obtained from the right ear of the patient described in Case 3 during session 2.

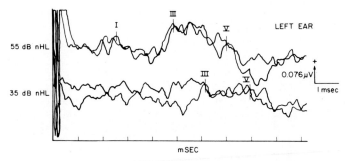

Figure 2-27. Click elicited BAER obtained from the left ear of the patient described in Case 3 during session 2.

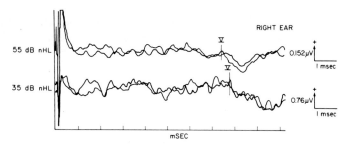

Figure 2-25. Click elicited BAER obtained from the right ear of the patient described in Case 3 during session 2.

Table 2-11 Click Latencies for Case 3

		Right	Left
Wave I	95 dB	1.67	1.78
	75 dB	2.01	no response
Wave III	95 dB	3.84	3.78
	75 dB	4.00	4.38
Wave V	95 dB	5.96	5.90
	75 dB	6.19	6.20
	55 dB	6.60	7.02
	35 dB	7.78	7.96

CASE 4

History

This 15-month-old male was referred to rule out a suspected hearing loss. At 13 months of age, a high fever developed that subsequently developed into viral meningitis and encephalitis. Prior to this time, the parents reported that the child responded appropriately to sound. Following his release from the hospital, the parents noted a marked deterioration in response to sounds and, essentially, an absence of any further development of speech and language.

Test Procedures

Initial testing consisted of immittance and BAER procedures. BAERs were elicited using clicks and tone bursts centered at 500, 1000, and 2000Hz, bilaterally.

Test Results

Type 2 tympanograms were obtained, bilaterally, but no acoustic reflexes could be elicited from either ear. Figures 2-28 through 2-30 depict the BAERs elicited from the right ear by clicks and tone bursts. No reliable responses could be elicited by either stimuli from the left ear. Absolute latencies of right ear data are shown in Table 2-12.

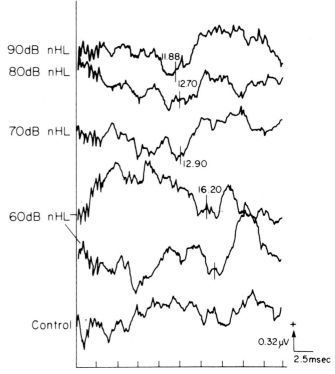

Figure 2-29. SN10 BAER to a 1000Hz tone burst obtained from the right ear of the patient described in Case 4.

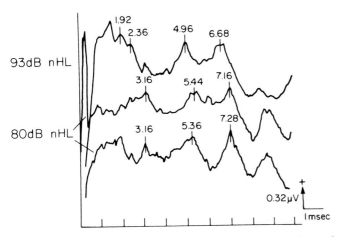

Figure 2-28. High-intensity, click elicited BAERs obtained from the right ear of the patient described in Case 4.

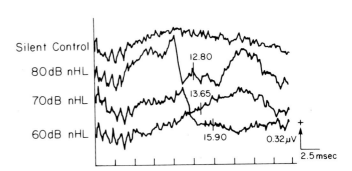

Figure 2-30. SN10 BAER elicited from the right ear of the patient described in Case 4, using a 2000Hz tone burst.

Table 2.12 Click Latencies for
Case 4

Wave	I	III	V
93 dB	2.36	4.96	6.68
80 dB	3.16/3.16*	5.44/5.36*	7.16/7.28*

* = Test-retest reliability

Based upon response morphology and amplitude, data at 80 dB were considered to be supra-threshold by approximately 10 dB. SN10 latencies are shown in Table 2-13.

Initial BAER techniques were administered when the patient was 15 months old. At 24 months of age, behavioral procedures were administered using operant techniques. No reliable responses could be obtained from the patient's left ear using behavioral procedures. A comparison of initial BAER thresholds with behavioral thresholds revealed the relationships described in Table 2-14.

Based upon immittance, acoustic reflex, and initial evoked potential data, a moderately powerful body aid was recommended for the right ear. Fitting was not changed based upon behavioral testing. The discrepancy between BAER and behavioral results at 500Hz was attributed to the reduced maximum power

Table 2.13 SN10
Latencies for Case 4

500Hz	no response
1000Hz	12.8 at 80 dB
	13.7 at 70 dB
	15.9 at 60 dB
2000Hz	11.9 at 90 dB
	12.7 at 80 dB
	12.9 at 70 dB
	16.2 at 60 dB

output (MPO) of the signal averager at this frequency. It should be noted that MPO will vary as a function of stimulus frequency and duration and that the examiner must be aware of instrumentation limitations at each test frequency.

This case demonstrates the major strength of evoked potential testing, namely the early detection of a hearing loss. Early detection allows the initiation of habilitative techniques at a much younger age than is otherwise possible, which should reduce the deleterious effects of a hearing loss on developing speech and language skills.

Table 2-14 Behavioral Thresholds for Case 4

		500Hz	1000Hz	2000Hz	Clicks
Right Ear	BAER	no response*	65 dB	60 dB	70 dB
	Behavioral	80 dB	60–70 dB	65 dB	—

* Intensity Limit of 75dB nHL at 500 Hz on our evoked potential equipment

SUMMARY

These 4 case studies demonstrate the types of responses that can be expected from patients of various ages and levels of auditory integrity. The major audiological benefit of the BAER techniques used is that it is possible to obtain threshold data from each ear at specific test frequencies at a much earlier age than is possible using behavioral procedures. These data are reliable and, based upon behavioral results, valid estimates of the patient's auditory sensitivity.

As with any physiological response, however, the test assesses the *functional integrity* of the auditory system and is not a direct measure of "hearing." While behavioral tests need not be administered to every patient who receives a physiologically based test, the examiner must not ignore the overall purpose of testing.

REFERENCES

Davis, H, Hirsh, SK (1979). A slow brainstem response for low frequency audiometry. *Audiology 18*, 445–461

Davis, H, Owen, JH (1985). Auditory evoked potentials. In JH Owen, & H Davis (Eds.), *Evoked potential testing:Clinical applications* (pp. 55–108). Orlando: Grune & Stratton

Feldman, AF & Wilbur, LA. Tympanometry Procedures, Interpretation, Variability. In AF Feldman & LA Wilbur (eds.), *The Measurement of Middle Ear Function*. Baltimore: Williams & Wilkins, 1976

Jewett, DL, Williston, JS (1971). Auditory-evoked far fields averaged from the scalp of humans. *Brain 94*, 681–696.

Owen, JH (1982). Influence of acquisition parameters on the reliability of the late auditory evoked response. *Clin EEG 13*, 85–86

Owen, JH, Davis, H (1985). *Evoked potential testing:Clinical applications*. Orlando: Grune & Stratton

Charles D. Donohoe

3

Application of the Brainstem Auditory Evoked Response in Clinical Neurologic Practice

Brainstem auditory evoked responses (BAER) have been the subject of numerous text and review articles. The purpose of this chapter is not to redescribe the history or technical aspects, but to present data. These untouched data are derived from patients with conditions representative of clinical neurologic practice. Corroborating information will include audiograms, computed tomographs (CT), and magnetic resonance images (MRI). These cases include the more common settings in which we have found the BAER to be useful. Realizing that many aspects remain controversial, the thoughts on interpretations, applications, and significance will be our own, as well as others in the literature. Audiologic factors will be stressed in that from a neurologic perspective their emphasis needs reinforcement.

At the outset, we would agree that all modalities of evoked potentials have been overused and applied in many situations where there is little chance of increasing diagnostic accuracy or directing therapy. The same may be said, however, of electroencephalography (EEG), electromyography (EMG), angiography, CT, and now MRI. Certainly valid clinical research has a different perspective and latitude compared with the situation in clinical practice, where a test should have proven relevant impact before the patient is exposed to the procedure and its expense. We believe a role does exist for the BAER in clinical neurologic practice when used on a selective basis and interpreted with a conservatism that arises from the realization that important neuroanatomic and neurophysiologic aspects of the procedure await elucidation (Fig. 3-1).

Following is a list of the five wave forms:

Wave I: peripheral portion of cranial nerve VIII adjacent to cochlea. Wave II: intracranial but extramedullary portion of cranial nerve VIII. Wave III: superior olivary nucleus. Others

claim the cochlear nucleus (Moller, 1983). Wave IV: lateral lemniscus. Wave V: inferior colliculus.

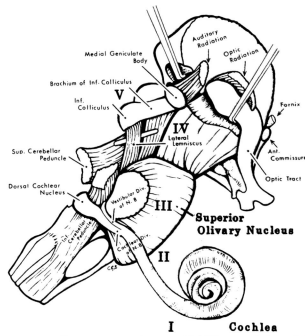

Figure 3-1.   Putative sites of origin of BAER waves I through V. From Smith, C.G. (1981). Serial dissection of the human brain. Baltimore-Munich: Urban & Schwarzenberg. p. 60. With permission.

Clinical Atlas of Auditory Evoked Potentials
ISBN 0-8089-1896-6

THE NORMAL BAER

The ability to determine a normal brainstem auditory evoked response is really the essence of familiarity with the procedure. Its foundation rests upon the recording of normative data and becoming accustomed to the variability under optimum conditions and in situations where ambient artifact degrades the expected response. Interpretation of these data implies an understanding of significant limitations of the procedure. It also realizes that the neurologic and audiologic influences are of inseparable importance. Traditionally, the interface between the disciplines of clinical neurology and audiology has been confined. It is the contention of our laboratory that the failure to scrutinize data without the perspective of routine audiologic principles is a most frequent and often a most embarrassing pitfall of BAER interpretation. Table 3-1 is a comparison of absolute latency values from various laboratories, including our own, studying normal adult subjects. This underscores the rather remarkable agreement of normative data between laboratories. Table 3-2 presents values for interpeak latencies, the primary criterion in neurologic interpretation. Tables 3-3 and 3-4 cite our acquisition parameters and norms separated on sex differences. Technique, sex of subject age and temperature can have significant impact on BAER latency and amplitude. (Fig. 3-2 A & B)

Table 3-2 Mean and Standard Deviation of Interpeak Latency Values from Several Laboratories

Investigation	N	I–III	III–V	I–V
Chiappa et al. (1979)	50	2.1 (.15)	1.9 (.16)	4.0 (.23)
Rowe (1978)	25	2.0 (.16)	2.0 (.20)	3.9 (.22)
Stockard & Rossiter (1977)	125	2.1 (.2)	1.9 (.2)	4.0 (.2)
Owen (1984)	34	2.1 (.24)	2.0 (.20)	4.2 (.20)

Standard deviations are given in parentheses.
N = number of patients in sample.
All values are given in milliseconds.

Table 3-3 Acquisition Parameters

Stimulus	Click
Level	65 dB SL
Polarity	Rarefaction
Time	1.0 mSec/Div
Sweeps	2000
Rate	11.4/Sec
Duration of click	100 μSec (microseconds)
Sensitivity	25 uV
Low Frequency Filter	150 Hz
High Frequency Filter	3000 Hz
Reference	Cz
Active	A1/A2
Ground	Fpz

Table 3-1 Comparison of Mean Absolute Latency for Each BAER Wave in a Study of Normal Adults

Investigation	N	Click Intensity	Filter (Hz)	Absolute Latency (msec)				
				I	II	III	IV	V
Rowe (1978)	25	60 dB	100–3000	1.9	2.9	3.8	5.1	5.8
Stockard et al. (1978)	50	60 dB	100–3000	1.8	2.9	3.9	5.2	5.8
Chiappa et al. (1979)	50	60 dB	100–3000	1.7	2.8	3.9	5.1	5.7
Owen (1984)	34	65 dB	150–3000	1.7	2.8	3.8	5.0	5.8

Table 3-4 Evoked Potential Data, age matched,
separated on basis of sex for both BAER and PSVER
(Pattern Shift Visual Evoked Response).

Brainstem Auditory Evoked Responses (all values are in msec)

	Wave	Mean	Mean + 3 SD		Mean	Mean + 3 SD
Men	I	1.65	2.04	Women	1.62	2.02
	III	3.79	4.21		3.74	4.10
	V	5.82	6.36		5.58	5.88
	I–III	2.14	2.65		2.12	2.60
	III–V	2.02	2.68		1.86	2.34
	I–V	4.16	4.82		3.97	4.33

Pattern Shift Visual Evoked Responses (all values in msec)

	Wave	Mean	Mean + 3 SD		Mean	Mean + 3 SD
Men	P100	98.3	114.5	Women	93.2	101.2

Normative data are frequently not separated on the basis of sex. As have other labs, we have found significant differences between men and women in latency values utilizing pattern shift VER and BAER.

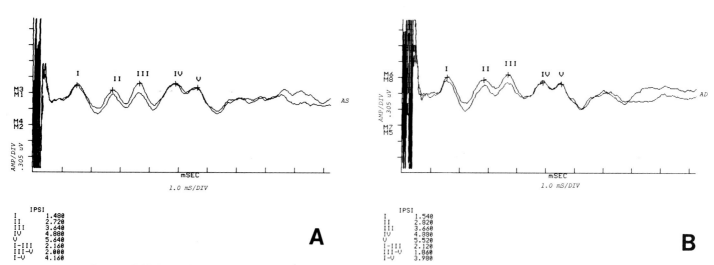

Figure 3-2. Case 1: BAERs with normal absolute and interpeak latency values. Ipsi refers to ipsilateral montage (Cz referred to the stimulated mastoid). (A) Normal BAER from left ear (AS) (B) Normal BAER from right ear (AD).

Case 1 (Fig. 3-2) is a representative normal BAER demonstrating easily identifiable wave forms. Case 2 (Fig. 3-3 A & B) illustrates the commonly occurring IV–V complex, of which there are multiple variations and the morphology of which can differ between ears of the same individual. The utility of the contralateral montage in differentiating waves IV and V is demonstrated.

Basic criteria and standards for recording have been the subject of several monographs. It is our experience that in the real world there is tremendous variability of acquisition parameters. In clinical use, there has also been an unfortunate practice of reporting results without presenting the actual wave forms. This totally eliminates the opportunity for another observer to confirm the findings. We support a format of documentation that cites the acquisition parameters and simultaneously presents ipsilateral and contralateral wave forms. This provides a check for the identification of the various elements of a response. In many normal as well as abnormal results, the designation of specific waves is frequently a debatable point. Unless the recorded waves can be scrutinized independently, a "blind" interpretation should be viewed with extreme skepticism.

Case 2

The IV–V Complex and the Value of the Contralateral Montage (Cz referred to contralateral mastoid) (Figs. 3-3 A & B).

Case 2 is presented to demonstrate the utility of the contralateral electrode pair in combination with the standard or ipsilateral pair (Cz referred to the stimulated mastoid). With the use of the contralateral placement, separation of waves IV and V is facilitated, the amplitude of wave III is reduced, and wave II is increased. In situations where morphology of waves is degraded, the simultaneous recording of the contralateral reference can aid in specific wave identification. Most commercially available machines have more than one channel and the inclusion of multiple electrode pairs is frequently beneficial in difficult cases. Wave I identification can sometimes be facilitated by the "horizontal" montage configuration (active electrode at contralateral mastoid and reference at stimulated mastoid).

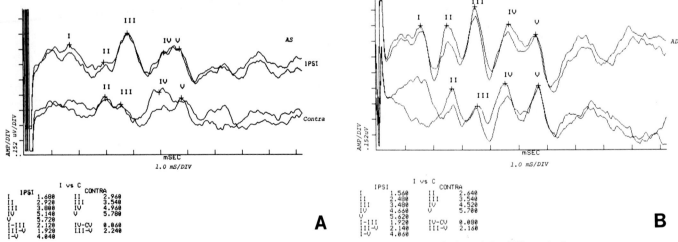

Figure 3-3. (A & B) Demonstrate value of contralateral montage (bottom trace in each figure) in differentiating component waves of BAER. Absolute and interpeak latencies of ipsilateral and contralateral montages are printed below traces (Case 2).

INTERPRETATION

There is no characteristic BAER abnormality that is specific to a particular neurologic lesion or disease. The principal pathologic findings in neurologic disease include abnormalities of the interpeak intervals that reflect conduction times from the peripheral end organ (wave I) to more central generators, wave III and wave V (see Fig. 3-1). This pathway is divided into the I–V, I–III, and III–V segments (Fig. 3-4). From a neurologic perspective, the use of these interpeak intervals is preferable in that it tends to reduce peripheral audiologic effects upon the interpretation and provides a modicum of localization as well. In the case of prolongation of the I–III interval, the abnormality could be placed between the cochlea and the lower pons. A classic example would be an acoustic neuroma. A prolongation of the III–V interwave interval would place the abnormality in the auditory tract between the lower pons and midbrain. A corresponding example is multiple sclerosis (MS).

Unfortunately, as is often the case in neurology, the simplicity and neatness of this approach is not always applicable in a clinical context. For example, in MS, a common situation in which the BAER is applied, most of the abnormalities are manifest by attenuation or absence of later waves. For example, a midbrain lesion may result in complete loss of waves IV and V, with intact earlier waves. In our experience as well as that of others (Chiappa et al., 1980), amplitude reduction of wave V is the most common BAER finding in individuals with MS who exhibit abnormal BAERs (about 30 percent of our total MS population). Normally, the wave V to wave I ratio exceeds 1. A ratio below 0.5 would be considered abnormal. It must be realized that these ratios vary at different intensity levels of stimulation and are influenced by hearing loss. In that regard, amplitude abnormalities are less reliable in neurologic use but may represent the only abnormal findings.

The cause of amplitude reductions is multifactorial and all interpretations should be based on a foundation of previous experience and conservative clinical correlation. This emphasizes the need for obtaining normative data and becoming familiar with results over varying conditions, such as temperature, montage and filter setting. We recommend criteria suggested by the American EEG Society for interpreting the BAER in clinical use. It should be noted that the response obtained must be reliable, which requires replication of traces and development of criteria for determining reliability. Though published norms can be used as initial guides, each laboratory should establish its own norms and practical experience. This includes the determination of cutoff values that are anticipated to distinguish normal from abnormal results. These values will give an indication of variance (standard deviation) and should provide a practical check of the procedural integrity of the system. Given a sample distribution of normal values, 68.3 percent of the sample values will fall within 1 standard deviation of the mean (normalized average). Ninety-five and one-half percent of the sample values will fall within 2 standard deviations, and 99.7 percent within three. We utilize 3 standard deviations in our determinations.

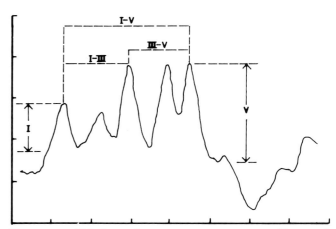

Figure 3-4. This figure demonstrates measurement of interpeak intervals I–III, I–V, III–V. These intervals serve as primary neurologic criteria in that they are less influenced by peripheral audiologic factors than are the absolute latencies or amplitudes of waves I, III or V.

Table 3-5 Various Methods that may Improve Specific
Identification of Waves I, III and V.

Wave I

1. Horizontal montage—relocate referential electrode to non-test ear. Improves wave I in about 1 in 6 cases. (see case #3 Fig. 3-5 A & C).

2. Use of external canal EEG needle electrode.

3. Use of nasopharyngeal electrode.

4. All waveforms can usually be improved by increasing stimulus intensity levels. When a large stimulus artifact occurs, the use of alternating polarity may improve wave I.

Wave III

1. Use of contralateral mastoid electrode. This will increase wave II, decrease wave III amplitude, and accentuate the separation between waves IV and V (see discussion of Case 2). (Fig. 3-3 A & B).

2. Repeated trials.

Wave V

1. Use of contralateral electrode. (Figs. 3-3 A & B)

2. Increased stimulus intensity. Excessive increases in stimulus intensity (e.g., 80–90 dB SL) are unnecessary and unpleasant for the patient. In addition, high-intensity stimulation alters the morphology of the IV–V complex so that the amplitude of wave IV exceeds that of wave V and measurement of intervals may be subject to error (see discussion of Case 3). (Fig. 3-5 b D).

3. Decreased stimulus intensity to a point where other waves become attenuated and only wave V remains.

4. Use of horizontal montage. If the wave considered to be wave V does not decrease in amplitude with this electrode placement, it is probably not wave V (see discussion of case 3). (Fig. 3-5 C).

A final word on interpretation concerns the importance of accurately identifying the waves used to determine interpeak measurements. Table 3-5 presents a variety of procedures worth trying to improve waves I, III, and V. Like most things, these procedures are not quite as easy as they appear. As with EEG and EMG, conservative interpretation (see Table 3-6) is the preferred course of action.

Table 3-6 Summary of Interpretation Criteria of the BAERs in Neurologic Practice.

1. Interpeak latency values I–III, III–V, I–V. These reduce peripheral audiologic influences.

2. Inter-aural differences between interpeak latencies. Values greater than 0.4 msec are abnormal in our lab.

3. Absence of waves or gross morphologic differences between ears.

4. Attenuation of waves. Wave V : Wave I ratio of less than 0.5 is considered abnormal. As a function of wave amplitude, this is less specific and is influenced by peripheral audiologic factors, intensity of stimulation, montage, temperature and acquisition parameters.

5. In many situations, wave I is difficult to identify limiting interpeak measurements. The basic nature of the system suggests that wave I does appear earlier than 1.4 msec. Using our norms of the I–V interpeak interval of 4.2 plus 3 standard deviations (0.2), 4.8 + 1.4 = 6.2 msec. If wave V occurs at or before 6.2 msec, there is probably nothing about the BAER indicative of a central (neurologic) abnormality. Little can be said of possible coexistent auditory pathology or inter-aural and amplitude changes.

Case 3 (Fig. 3-5 A and B)

The effects of electrode placement and increased stimulus intensity upon the BAER are depicted in figure 3-5 (A–E). (A) A well-formed BAER with the IV–V complex at an intensity of 60 dB SL. (B) Contralateral montage that increases the separation between waves IV and V and decreases the amplitude of wave III. (C) Horizontal montage—note the increase in wave I and the disap-pearance of wave V. (D) These are data from the same patient, utilizing an increased stimulus intensity of 85 dB SL. Note that wave IV becomes larger than wave V, which is difficult to identify. (E) This is the contralateral montage at high-level-intensity stimulation, which once again demonstrates the separation between wave IV and wave V.

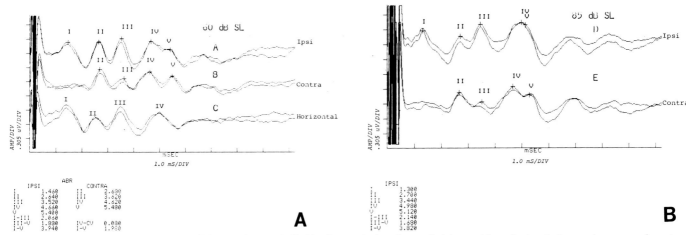

Figure 3-5. (A & B) BAER from (right) ear of same individual recorded under varied intensities of stimulation and montage locations (A thru E) (Case 3).

EFFECTS OF PERIPHERAL AUDITORY DYSFUNCTION UPON THE BAER

Laboratories utilizing the BAER have tended to evolve into those using it for primary audiologic and those using it for primary neurologic purposes. This separation is artificial and it is important to understand the effects of abnormalities of the peripheral auditory system upon the central pathways. Generally, the discipline of clinical neurology tends to place rather weak emphasis on audiologic principles. The purpose of this section is to review the changes of both conductive and sensorineural (SN) hearing loss upon the BAER. Before those details, it is essential to recognize that the psychological event we term "hearing" is not directly measured by the BAER, and normal BAERs have been seen in both the cortically deaf and in anencephalic infants (Hecox, 1983). Rather we are monitoring neuronal components in the peripheral and central auditory tract. Consistent with that is the variance of the BAERs in patients with very similar audiometric configurations.

Hearing losses are generally divided into conductive and SN. Conductive losses occur when sound cannot reach the cochlea. This blockage may be secondary to abnormalities of the canal, the eardrum, and the ossicles, including the foot plate of the stapes. Examples of conductive loss would include foreign bodies within the external canal, maldevelopment of the external ear (Treacher-Collins syndrome), otosclerosis (the most common conductive loss in the 15–50 year age group), and infections such as serous otitis media in children. Conductive hearing loss reduces the effective stimulus reaching the cochlea. The latency of BAER component waves is prolonged, in patients with conductive impairment, by an amount commensurate to the hearing loss. Utilizing the latency of wave V versus click intensity, a characteristic shift from the normal curve can be determined (see Fig. 3-6).

In conductive loss, the amount of shift gives a fair estimate of the patient's hearing loss (see discussion Fig. 3-7 A & B). For example, when a 60 dB HL click is used to evoke a BAER in a patient with a 40 dB conductive hearing loss, only 20 dB reaches the cochlea, and the corresponding latency would approach that of a 20 dB SL click stimulus. In other words, the patient's latency-intensity function for a given BAER would parallel the normal but would be displaced in time. When an impairment is unilateral, the inter-aural difference of wave V will be increased. It is for that reason in neurologic use that stimuli should be referenced to sensation levels of the specific individual (dB SL) rather than to hearing levels of a normal adult population (dB HL). The use of interpeak interval measurements will reduce audiologic influences. Practical difficulties in identifying wave forms (such as wave I) do exist, however, and common pathologic conditions cause disappearance of multiple waves, further limiting the application of interpeak intervals as the sole diagnostic criteria.

SN hearing loss occurs when the cochlea or eighth nerve is damaged. This may occur on a hereditary basis, or may be post-traumatic, post-infectious (i.e., mumps), or may occur as a consequence of drug toxicity. Noise-induced hearing loss is the most common and most important of the occupational impairments. Exposure to industrial noise levels greater than 90 dB for months or years can cause significant cochlear damage. Other commonly encountered SN-type losses would be the situation in Meniere's disease, which results in fluctuating hearing loss involving the low-frequency tones. As the disease progresses, the hearing loss becomes greater, involving all tones, and may eventually become total. Recruitment of loudness is commonly demonstrated. The acoustic neuroma is a rare cause of SN loss but its importance to clinical neurology is obvious. Regarding the interpretation of the BAER, the effects of hearing loss cannot be overstated. To place the situation in perspective, it is estimated that more than 16,000,000 Americans suffer significant auditory loss.

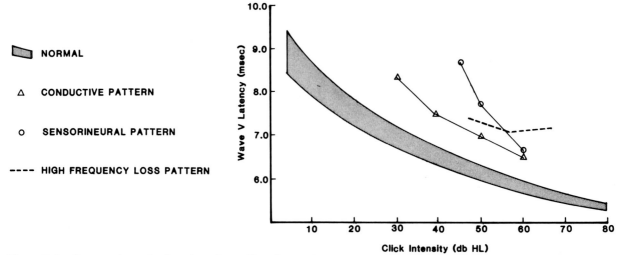

Figure 3-6. Latency-intensity function of wave V under conditions of normal hearing as well as conductive, sensorineural and high frequency loss.

The presence of a SN hearing loss has more complex ramifications than does a conductive loss upon the BAER. Reduction in wave I amplitude is more common than in the conductive loss. (See discussion Case 5, Fig. 3-8) When SN impairment is unilateral, inter-aural absolute wave V differences have been reported to increase by as much as 1.5 msec. In patients with unilateral SN loss greater than 50 dB at 4000Hz, latency-intensity functions are more variable but usually exhibit an abruptly steeper slope in the middle-intensity range. The exact form of the curve may depend on whether the loss is predominantly high-frequency (such as a noise-induced impairment) or is more equally distributed in nature. In general, SN-impaired patients with flat audiometric configurations have prolonged wave V latencies in response to low-intensity clicks. As the energy level of the stimulus is increased, the latency decreases to near-normal values. The slope of the latency-intensity function increases sharply as threshold is approached. This phenomenon has been associated with loudness recruitment.

In patients with precipitous SN hearing loss, a wave V latency-intensity function can be seen that may be difficult to distinguish from a conductive loss (Fria, 1980). This may relate to cochlear mechanics and the organization of hair cells in apical regions of the basilar membrane. In conclusion, conductive and SN impairments can differentially alter the BAER, and awareness of this problem is necessary in clinical neurologic use.

It is recognized that the standard click used in the BAER represents a spectrum of frequencies, and patients with strictly low-frequency hearing loss below 1500Hz can be overlooked using click evoked threshold responses. Another group of hearing losses that can be missed are those involving 4000Hz and above. In general, the use of click evoked responses primarily evaluates the integrity of the peripheral auditory apparatus between 1500 and 4000Hz. When utilizing the click to evaluate auditory sensitivity, it should be remembered that a normal threshold can be found in the face of a hearing loss involving either the high or low frequencies. This loss can have distinct effects upon the BAER and its proper interpretation (see discussion of Fig. 3-9 A,B,C, case 6).

CONDUCTIVE HEARING LOSS

Case 4

This seven-year-old boy exhibited moderate psychomotor retardation with autistic features. He was nonverbal until age six. He had a history of multiple ear infections and because of behavioral problems could not be evaluated audiometrically using standard procedures. The BAER at various intensity levels of stimulation (40, 55, and 75 dB nHL) exhibits the latency-intensity shift of waves I and V characteristic of a conductive hearing loss (Figs. 3-7 A & B). In general, the latencies of the waves are shifted in time to a degree commensurate with the hearing loss. Although the wave I absolute latency at low levels of stimulation is prolonged, it is well-formed and easily identifiable. When it is difficult to establish threshold levels (dB SL), the latency shift produced by a conductive loss could be subject to misinterpretation as a central abnormality, particularly if wave I is misidentified. The interpeak latencies remain normal in a conductive loss.

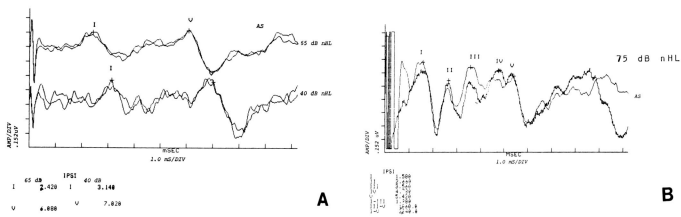

Figure 3-7. (A & B) BAER, left ear, of patient in case #4 demonstrating latency shift of waves I & V at increasing levels of stimulation, 40, 55 & 75 dB nHL (Case 4).

SENSORINEURAL HEARING LOSS

Case 5

This 60-year-old white male was referred for a BAER because of bilateral tinnitus and vertigo. CT scan of the brain was normal. The patient's auditory threshold using clicks was elevated at 40 dB nHL. Latency-intensity function was consistent with sensorineural hearing loss with poorly formed waves I and II and rather well formed waves III and V with normal absolute latencies (Fig. 3-8). A variety of techniques used to improve wave I were not successful. The difficulty in identifying wave I limits the utility of the I–III and I–V interpeaks. In our experience, in the face of a sensorineural hearing loss there is extreme variability in BAER morphology that does not correlate well with the magnitude of the hearing loss. Difficulties in identifying wave I are a particularly frequent problem.

EFFECT OF HIGH-FREQUENCY HEARING LOSS UPON BAER MORPHOLOGY

Case 6

This 22-year-old male was referred for a BAER because of persistent lightheadedness and disequilibrium following a rather trivial head injury. Neurologic exam, computed tomography, and electronystagmography (ENG) were all normal. A distinct difference is noted in the morphology of the BAER in the right versus the left ear (Fig. 3-9 A & B). The left ear (Fig. 3-9 A) morphology shows profound reduction in amplitude and absence of waves II, III, and IV, although the absolute and interpeak latencies of I and V remain within normal range. Threshold levels to the standard click were within 10 dB bilaterally. The audiogram is presented in Figure 3-9 C and reveals a high-frequency hearing loss with a sharp dropoff in the left ear above 4000Hz. The case is presented to demonstrate that the click stimulus best correlates with the audiogram between 2000 and 4000Hz, and above that level significant hearing loss can be present that will not be identified by click evoked threshold responses. In that regard, it is important to recognize that BAER morphologic changes of a significant degree can be predicated on a high-frequency hearing loss that may go unrecognized utilizing the standard click. In difficult situations, it is usually worthwhile to perform formal audiometric studies.

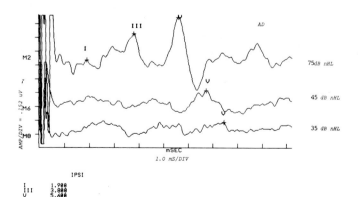

Figure 3-8. BAER at increasing levels of stimulation, 35, 45, 75 dB nHL in an individual with a sensorineural hearing loss (Case 5).

BAERs IN MULTIPLE SCLEROSIS

Multiple sclerosis has been recognized for more than 100 years. Despite massive scientific investigation that has revealed new facets of electrophysiology and epidemiology, the specifics regarding the nature of the disease and its proper treatment remain a mystery. Traditionally, multiple sclerosis has been regarded as the most important of the demyelinating disorders. It is the loss of myelin that interferes with normal saltatory conduction and produces a conduction block. Conductive slowing can also occur without clinical symptomatology. The demyelinating process and resultant abnormal modes of impulse conduction are influenced by multiple factors in the ambient milieu. Changes in temperature, pH, and ionic homeostasis, due to alterations produced by gliosis and edema of the white matter, may all play important contributing roles. Clinical practices suggest that the reasons for sudden deterioration in a patient are multifactorial and are not necessarily predicated on extension of underlying structural disease. With relevance to evoked potentials, it has been suggested that the disease process in MS is not limited to central nervous system (CNS) myelin, but that the peripheral nervous system may also be involved (Eisen et al., 1982).

It is well known that the frequency of the BAER in detecting silent lesions is far less than that of either the visual or somatosensory evoked potentials in all categories of MS. Explanations for this finding have included the fact that only a short segment of the brainstem is analyzed with this procedure, in contrast to the analysis of longer tracks with both the visual and somatosensory modalities. As with the visual evoked response, many BAER abnormalities in MS occur in subclinical disease states. Compared with the visual and somatosensory modalities, abnormalities in the BAER are uncovered approximately one-third as frequently in MS.

In MS there is a rather low incidence of pure-tone audiometric defects. However, inter-aural auditory delay can be abnormal at a given tone frequency even though the configuration of the audiogram is normal. Definite inter-aural delays have been demonstrated in patients whose thresholds for the left and right ear were similar to within 5 decibels (Regan, 1981). Similar situations exists in regard auditory stereo-acuity. The lower yield, in multiple sclerosis, of the BAER versus other tests may be a complex issue that is based upon parallel circuitry and the testing circumstances, where the simple click used to evoke a response tends to stress predominantly the higher frequencies. Neural signals representative of different tone frequencies may be spatially organized and delays restricted to one or more limited bands of tone would not be sampled by current methodology.

When abnormal in MS, BAERs tend to show absence of later wave components, attenuation of later waves, and increase in the interpeak intervals, particularly III–V. This is frequently a unilateral abnormality. The most common pattern that we have seen is amplitude reductions, particularly in wave V, but in wave IV as well. This type of abnormality is not at all particular to MS and occurs in a variety of diseases affecting brainstem white matter, such as leukoencephalopathies, polioencephalo-

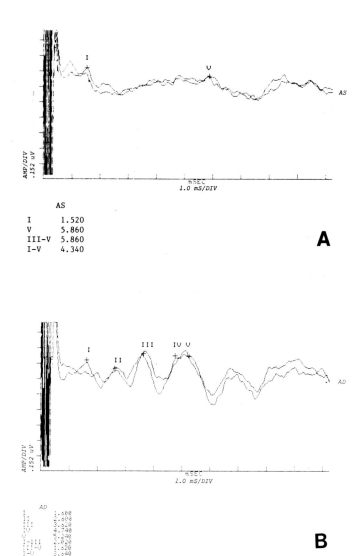

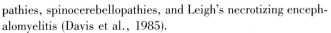

AS

I	1.520
V	5.860
III-V	5.860
I-V	4.340

A

AD

I   1.600
II   2.600
III 3.020
IV   4.740
V   5.240
I-III 1.420
III-V 1.020
I-V 3.640

B

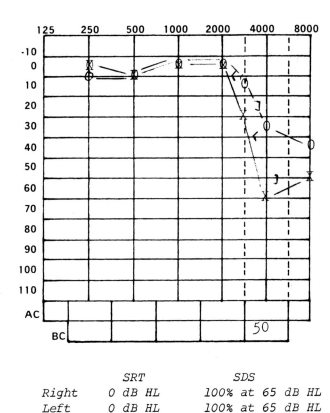

	SRT	SDS
Right	*0 dB HL*	*100% at 65 dB HL*
Left	*0 dB HL*	*100% at 65 dB HL*

C

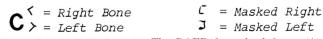

< = Right Bone   ⊏ = Masked Right
> = Left Bone   ⊐ = Masked Left

Figure 3-9. (A,B,C) Case 6. The BAER from the left ear (A) shows a reduction in amplitude and disruption of normal BAER component waves as compared with right ear (B). (C) Audiogram (ANSF, 1969) of same patient with sharp drop off in left ear in high frequency range (400Hz). Note: If there is an unexplained inter-aural morphologic difference in the BAER, electrode impedance levels should always be checked as well (Case 6).

pathies, spinocerebellopathies, and Leigh's necrotizing encephalomyelitis (Davis et al., 1985).

The low yield with BAER testing in MS does not eliminate its utility in objectively evaluating clinical symptoms such as dizziness, unsteadiness, and disequilibrium. This raises a point of controversy regarding the ultimate justification of the expense and effort exerted in diagnosing a disease such as multiple sclerosis that has no specific cure. We find these criticisms to be shallow in light of the patient's dilemma as that patient wrestles with symptoms that go unexplained and that frequently provoke psychological explanations from physicians. Our experience with MS is that many patients are initially given primary psychiatric diagnoses and are exposed to all the frustration and confusion that this mistake carries with it.

As magnetic resonance imaging (MRI) becomes increasingly available, so does the tremendous promise it holds in neuro-diagnosis. It is frequently the tendency of neurologists and physicians in general to be most impressed with that which they can see. The meandering wave form of the VER and BAER certainly evokes a less dramatic impact than does the sagittal section of the human brain, on MRI. From a standpoint of practical neurology, the ability to provide insight into the presence of demyelinating disease is most critical early in the disorder, before clinical signs become very characteristic. Whether magnetic resonance will assume a pre-eminent role in the confirmation of early MS remains a question. It is our preliminary sense of this issue that leads us to believe additional refinements beyond current MRI techniques will be necessary to achieve this goal.

A final note regarding multiple sclerosis concerns the BAER's role in monitoring a variety of therapies purportedly useful in that disease. Once again, we stress that there is an important difference between clinical practice and valid clinical research. In our own experience and that of others (Aminoff et al., 1984), this modality of evoked potential has not been a reliable indicator of disease state. In clinical practice, we see no justification for monitoring currently available therapies, such as high-dose steroids or immunosuppressives, utilizing evoked potentials as objective markers.

DEMYELINATING DISEASE

Case 7

This 42-year-old female (Fig. 3-10, A,B,C) complained to her obstetrician of progressive urgency of urination, numbness in her finger tips, and a "waddling" gait. CT was normal. Pattern shift visual evoked responses (PSVEP) (Fig. 3-10 C) showed prolonged latencies with P 100s at 145 and 151 msec. The BAER was abnormal on the left side (Fig. 3-10 A) with prolongation of the left III–V interpeak latency. Subsequent MRI, clinical course, and CSF studies have confirmed multiple sclerosis. The unilateral nature of the BAER abnormality is common (approximately 50 percent) in multiple sclerosis. In our experience, rather than subtle interpeak changes, the more frequent abnormality in multiple sclerosis is attenuation or absence of waves IV and V.

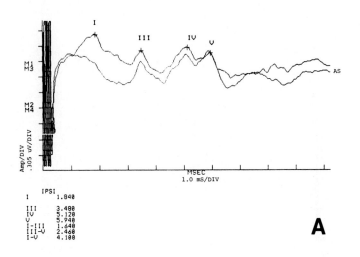

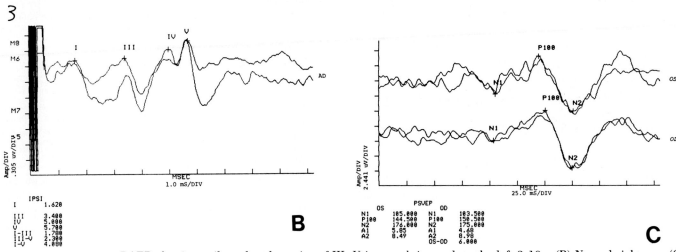

Figure 3-10. (A,B,C) BAER showing unilateral prolongation of III–V interpeak interval on the left 3-10a. (B) Normal right ear. (C) Visual evoked response is prolonged in both right and left eyes (OD and OS) (Case 7).

Case 7A

These BAERs in Figures 3-11 A,B,C,D were obtained from a 33-year-old cousin of the patient described in Case 7. Case 7A developed definite MS.

BAERs obtained over a 1-year interval show a characteristic progression from normal wave forms in 1984 (Figs. 3-11 A,B) to attenuation of waves IV and V, on the left (Fig. 3-11 C) and prolongation of the III–V interpeak interval on the right (Fig. 3-11 D) in 1985.

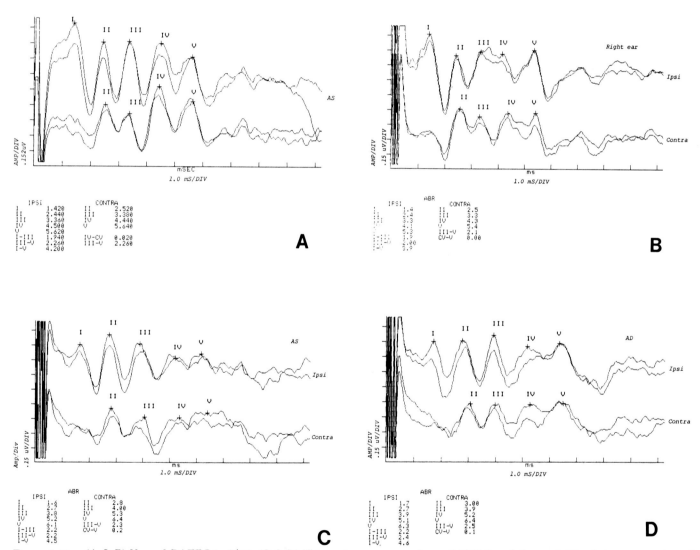

Figure 3-11. (A & B) Normal BAERS in 2/84. (C & D) This patient, one year later. BAER from left ear, 3-11c shows attenuation of later waves (IV & V). Right ear, 3-11d shows prolongation of III–V interval. Both changes are characteristic of MS (Case 7A).

Case 8

This 30-year-old white female presented to an emergency room with diplopia, numbness of her tongue, and truncal and appendicular ataxia. CT and pattern shift visual evoked response were normal. The BAER shows gross distortion of morphology with absence of waves IV and V on the left side and absence of wave V on the right. (Fig. 3-12 A,B) MRI demonstrated multiple areas of "increased signal" consistent with demyelinating disease. (Fig. 3-12 C,D,E) Spinal fluid analysis and clinical course were consistent with multiple sclerosis.

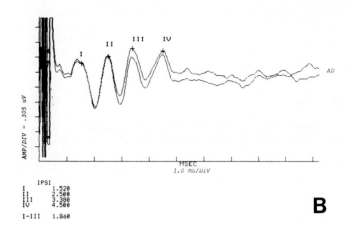

	IPSI
I	1.520
II	2.500
III	3.380
IV	4.500
I-III	1.860

B

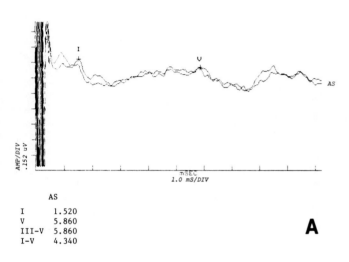

	AS
I	1.520
V	5.860
III-V	5.860
I-V	4.340

A

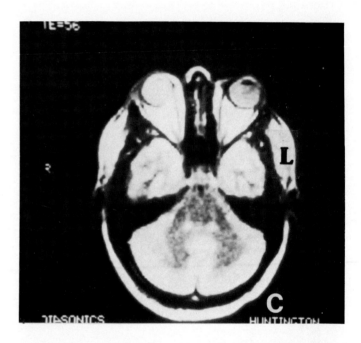

C

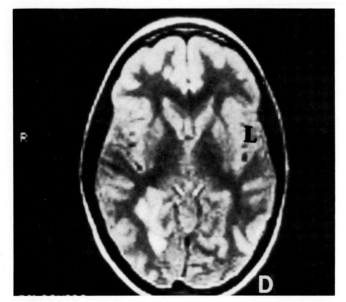

D

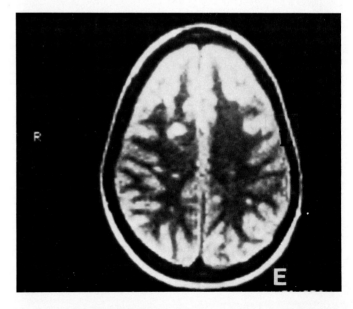

E

Figure 3-12. (A & B) BAER from left ear (A) exhibits absence of waves IV & V. Right ear (B) exhibits absence of wave V. These are the most common findings in MS. (C & E) MRI scans demonstrate multiple areas of increased signal on T 2 weighted images (Case 8).

Case 9

This 32-year-old white female was evaluated for a 1-year history of facial numbness, dysarthria, and progressive ataxia. At the time that these BAERs were performed, her clinical symptomatology was of mild to moderate severity. Visual evoked responses were abnormal bilaterally. MRI scan showed multiple areas of increased signal within the white matter, consistent with demyelinating disease. (Fig. 3-13 C,D) BAERs show well-formed waves I and II, but beyond that there is profound desynchronization and identification of later waves (beyond wave II) is difficult. (Fig. 3-13 A,B) We find this case to be of value in its relationship to MS, but also of interest regarding cerebral death. Indeed, we have an individual who has only moderate clinical involvement, but it is hard to identify any waves beyond waves I and II. Her audiogram was normal. It has been suggested that disappearance of all waves other than I and II is a consistent pattern with cerebral death. We feel that this pattern can occur with demyelinating disease of even a mild to moderate clinical degree. The possibility of unrecognized pre-existent conditions such as MS poses a rare but significant dilemma, and reduces the utility of the BAER in cerebral death determinations. A final point is that despite the severely abnormal BAER, the MRI image of the brainstem appears normal but the paraventricular white matter shows multiple obvious areas of increased signal.

THE USE OF THE BAER IN ACOUSTIC NEUROMAS

Acoustic neuromas (schwannomas) account for approximately 5 percent of all intracranial neoplasms. They are the most common tumor of the cerebellopontine angle, representing about 80 percent of the lesions in this area. Meningiomas (5 percent), cholesteatomas (5 percent), dermoids (5 percent), and a variety of other lesions (abscesses, arachnoid cysts) are much less frequent in this locale. Bilateral acoustic neuromas are usually seen in the setting of neurofibromatosis.

Unilateral hearing loss, tinnitus, and disequilibrium are the most common clinical symptoms of acoustic neuromas. An individual with a unilateral sensorineural hearing loss and tinnitus is an immediate suspect for such a lesion. (See Table 3-7) Although in an overall perspective, acoustic neuromas represent a rare cause of SN hearing loss (less than 1 percent of cases), an

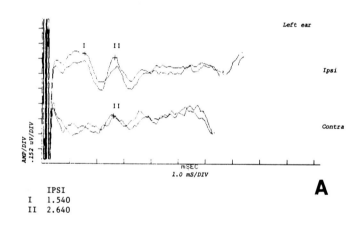

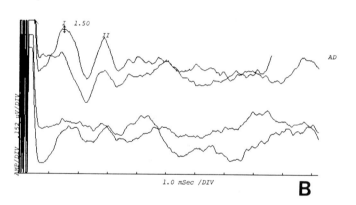

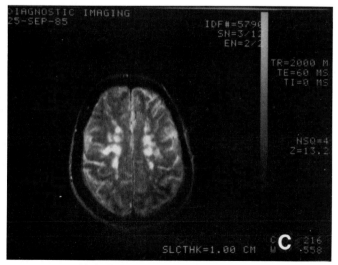

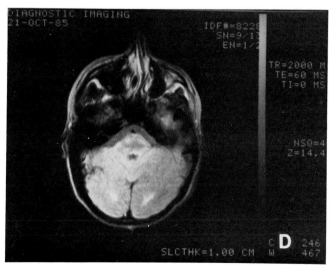

Figure 3-13. (A & B) Severely abnormal BAERs in both ears with no recognition of waves beyond wave II. 3-13c & d: MRI scan shows multiple areas of increased signal in the periventricular white matter (C), but no abnormalities are identified in brainstem (D) (Case 9).

individual whose hearing loss is such that speech discrimination is unduly poor in comparison with the ability to hear pure tones should prompt an even higher index of suspicion. CT scanning and now magnetic resonance imaging have proven to be highly effective modes of radiologic confirmation. With the advent of MRI, there has been improvement in the evaluation of the posterior fossa, particularly in eliminating bony artifact that hindered CT evaluation of that area. MRI, with the addition of surface coil and sequencing technology that improves the signal-to-noise performance and decreases slice thickness, will, it is hoped, provide a totally noninvasive modality for imaging the cerebellopontine angle and the internal auditory canal. At the time of this writing, these issues show rapid progress.

In general, tumors involving the cerebellopontine angle are associated with increases in the latency of all BAER component waves. The latencies of waves II through V are generally increased more than is that of wave I. This results in an increase in the interwave intervals I–III and I–V. Previously, the focus had assumed a more simplistic approach, using inter-aural absolute wave V latency differences greater than 0.3 msec as significant. Our own mean plus 3 standard deviations is 0.5 msec. It is important to realize, however, that the use of inter-aural absolute wave V differences as a primary criterion is not acceptable (Chiappa and Yiannikas, 1983). These wave V changes would be difficult to interpret with bilateral lesions but, more important, the utility of this measurement is distinctly limited in the face of profound hearing loss. This contrasts with the use of the interpeak interval measurements that are generally resistant to the effects of hearing loss. The point assumes considerable practicality in that in the series with which we are most familiar, the average hearing loss in almost 98 patients with acoustic neuroma approached 60 dB.

Another issue is that the I–V interpeak latency can be normal despite a prolonged I–III. This emphasizes that the system in question is not truly linear and that parallel circuitry can occur. Although prolongation of the I–III interpeak interval tends to be the most specific finding, experience in our own practice, as well as that of a surgical colleague who has removed 98 acoustic tumors, is somewhat different. We have both found that the BAER abnormalities in more than 50 percent of the cases shows gross disruption of all waves beyond wave I. In many of our cases, the ability to measure interpeak intervals I–III and I–V is not possible. This gross distortion of wave forms does not appear to be related either to tumor size or to hearing loss. In our experience, as well as that of our surgical colleague, the BAER has been abnormal in all patients with an acoustic neuroma (52/52 cases). Others suggest that on rare occasions the BAER can be normal in the face of an acoustic tumor, particularly a small intracanalicular lesion (Eggermont et al., 1986).

Information derived from intraoperative monitoring of cerebellopontine angle tumors in human patients and from observations in experimental dog models, suggests a sensitivity of the BAER to traction on the cerebellar hemisphere or the cochlear nerve (Sekiya et al., 1985) (Fig. 3-15). In this setting, it was

Table 3-7 Characteristic Audiologic Findings in Acoustic Neuroma

1. Unilateral sensorineural hearing impairment in 90 percent (almost three-fourths exhibit high-frequency involvement).

2. Impaired speech discrimination in 90 percent.

3. Absent acoustic reflex or reflex decay in 85 percent.

4. Reduced vestibular response (greater than 20 percent reduction on ENG) in 80 percent.

5. Absence of recruitment.

noticeable that the wave I peak remained stationary but that there was progressive latency prolongation and amplitude decrement of all waves beyond wave I. This suggests a conduction block between the extracranial portion of the cochlear nerve and the brainstem. This would agree with the I–III and I–V interwave interval changes seen in the clinical BAER. The situation in which all waves beyond wave I are degraded (the more common in our experience) may be a matter of degree. Another issue is the obliteration of all BAER components including wave I. Observation of these animal experiments, supported by neuropathologic studies in humans, suggests that this cannot be caused by a conduction block, but rather is a result of occlusion of the internal auditory artery.

Case 10

This 67-year-old female complained of numbness about the right side of her tongue and the roof of her mouth. She was unaware of any hearing loss, but upon formal audiometric studies there was a demonstrated 50 dB hearing loss on the right involving the high-frequency tones. The BAER on the left side was normal. (Fig. 3-14 A) On the right side, the response was severely degraded, including all waves and even the preservation of wave III is debatable. (Fig. 3-14 B) CT and subsequent surgery confirmed a large right acoustic neuroma. (Fig. 3-14 C,D) In our experience, this obvious disruption of wave form morphology is more common than are subtle interpeak latency changes. This obliteration of the BAER has not been solely dependent upon the degree of hearing loss (see discussion Figs. 3-15 A,B).

Figures 3-15 A,B demonstrate the changes on the evoked action potentials from the internal auditory meatus portion of the cochlear nerve (IAM-EAP) and the brainstem auditory evoked response (BAER) during manipulation of the cerebellopontine angle. Traction at this site produces marked prolongation of the I–V interpeak latency and amplitude decrement of waves II through V, but not of wave I. The obliteration of all BAER components, including wave I, is considered to be predicated on a vascular basis with secondary autolysis of the cochlear apparatus. BAER changes in the face of an acoustic neuroma frequently show severe morphologic disruption that may be predicated upon the effects of eighth-nerve traction and ultimate mechanical distortion of the relationship between the anterior inferior cerebellar (AICA) and the internal auditory arteries.

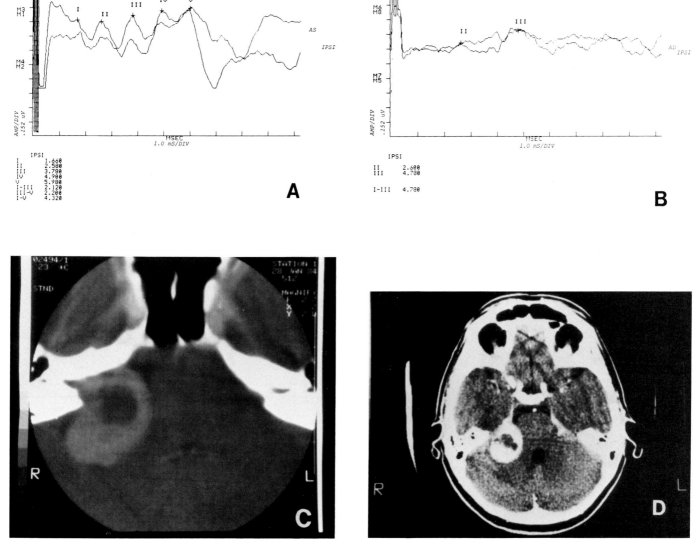

Figure 3-14. (A & B) Normal BAER on left. BAER on right (acoustic neuroma) is severely attenuated. Identification of any wave is debatable. (C & D) CT scan of large right acoustic neuroma (Case 10).

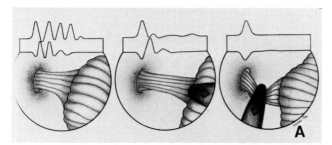

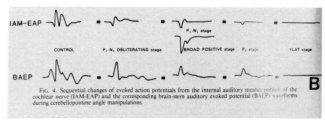

Figure 3-15. (A & B) Sequential changes of evoked action potentials from the internal auditory meatus portion of the cochlear nerve (IAM-EAP) and the corresponding brainstem auditory evoked response (BAER) waveforms during cerebellopontine angle manipulations. From Sekiya, T & Iwabuchi, T, & Kamata, S, *et al.* (1985). Deterioration of auditory evoked potentials during cerebellopontine angle manipulations. *J. Neurosurg, 63,* 599–602. With permission.

Case 11

This 39-year-old white female had been followed by an otolaryngologist for several years. Suddenly, in September of 1985, she noted a rather abrupt deterioration of her hearing in the left ear. Audiologic studies are presented in Figure 3-16 C. CT scan revealed a small, 1-cm lesion in the left cerebellopontine angle (Fig. 3-16 D,E). The BAER was normal on the right (Fig. 3-16 B), but the left side showed definite prolongation of the I–III as well as the I–V interpeak latencies, with marked inter-aural differences (Fig. 3-16 A). Surgery confirmed the presence of an acoustic neuroma. Although prolongation of the interpeak I–III interval is a characteristic finding in acoustic neuroma, our experience has been that the morphology of the BAER undergoes degradation and that frequently measurement of these interpeak intervals is not possible. The degree of these morphologic changes has not been related solely to hearing loss or tumor size.

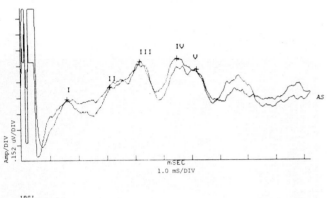

A

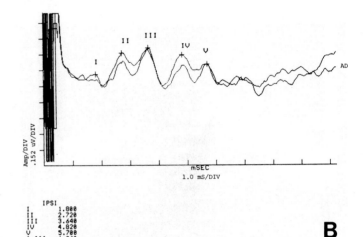

B

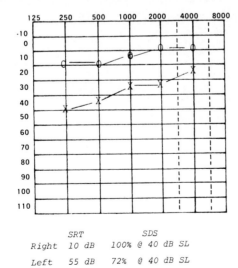

	SRT	SDS
Right	10 dB	100% @ 40 dB SL
Left	55 dB	72% @ 40 dB SL

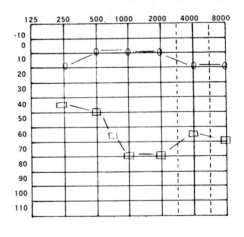

X = Right   Λ = Masked Right
O = Left   U = Masked Left

C

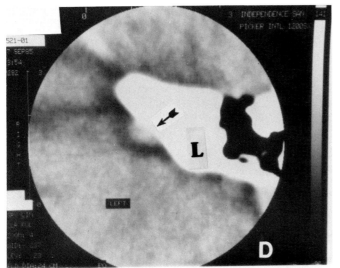
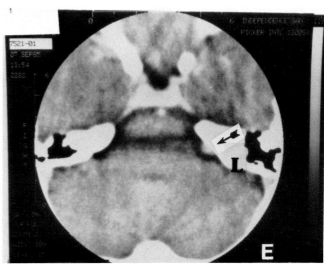

Figure 3-16. (A & B) BAER from 9/85 is normal on the right. On the left ear there is prolongation of the I–III and I—V interpeak intervals with a inter-aural prolongation of the left I–III of 0.72 msec greater than the right I–III. (values above 0.4 msec are considered abnormal). (C) Audiogram from 9/82 and 9/85 documenting magnitude of hearing loss. (D & E) CT scan of small (1 cm.) acoustic neuroma at internal acoustic meatus (see arrow) (Case 11).

RULING OUT ACOUSTIC NEUROMA

Case 12

This 32-year-old female complained of a 3-month history of fullness in the left ear, tinnitus, and episodic vertigo. CT (Fig. 3-17 C) was interpreted as suggestive of enlargement of the left internal auditory meatus and a soft tissue mass was suspected in the left cerebellopontine (CPA) angle. Both BAER (Fig. 3-17 A & B) and MRI were normal. The patient was considered not to have an acoustic neuroma (Fig. 3-17 D). This is representative of a situation where the ability to cross-check abnormalities suggested by other neurodiagnostic methods is helpful.

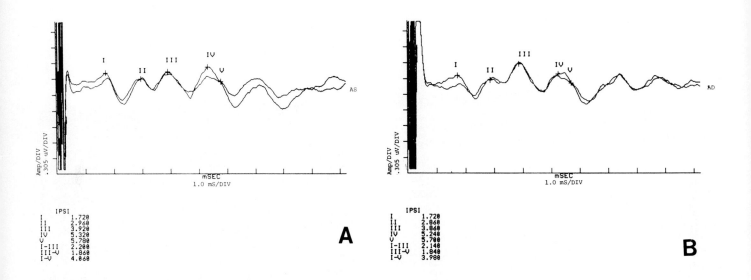

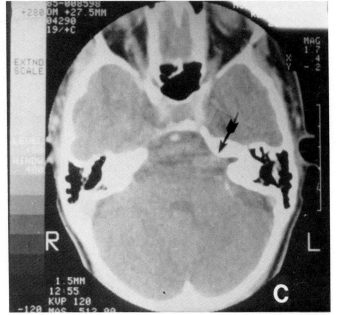

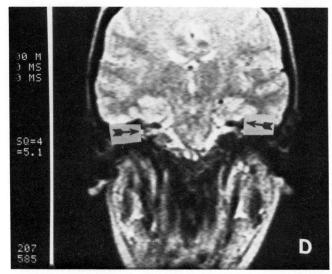

Figure 3-17.   (A & B) Normal BAERs from left (A) and right (B) ears. (C) CT scan interpreted as 'possible' left cerebellopontine angle tumor (see arrow). (D) Normal MRI scan (Case 12).

CEREBELLOPONTINE ANGLE LESION NOT ASSOCIATED WITH THE EIGHTH NERVE

Case 13

The patient is a 40-year-old male who presented with severe lancinating left facial pain and left hemifacial spasm. Tegretol controlled both symptoms. CT (Fig. 3-18 C) revealed a low-density lesion in the left cerebellopontine angle extending into the region of Meckel's cave. The BAER on the right side is normal. (Fig. 3-18 B) BAER on the left side (Fig. 3-18 A) shows prolongation of the I–III and I–V interwave latencies as compared to the right. He refused surgery. The neuroradiologic diagnosis was epidermoid tumor with subarachnoid cyst less likely. In our experience, lesions of the cerebellopontine angle not involving the eighth nerve generally do not produce the gross wave form disruption that is quite commonly seen in the acoustic neuromas.

UTILITY OF THE BAER IN THE COMATOSE STATE

A considerable literature exists purporting the efficacy of the BAER both in the determination of cerebral death and also

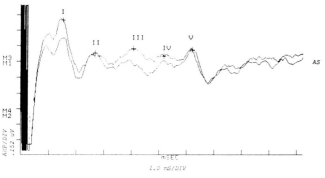

A

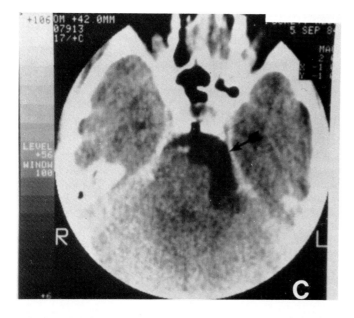

C

as a prognostic indicant in coma. It is our feeling that the determination of cerebral death rests on clinical grounds and that neurophysiologic studies, including the electroencephalogram (EEG) and multimodality evoked responses, assume a complementary but not an essential role in that diagnosis. A more controversial area is the ability to prognosticate both survival and quality of survival in individuals who are comatose for a variety of reasons, including trauma, post-hypoxic states, metabolic abnormalities, hemorrhage, and other insults to the central nervous system. Refinements to the clinical neurologic exam have certainly added to our understanding of physiologic conditions that, when present, imply an ultimate inability to sustain life (cerebral death). A problem continues to exist in predicting survival and ultimate outcome in individuals who are comatose but do not meet the criteria for cerebral death.

The ability to prognosticate in cases of cerebral injury using multimodality evoked potentials has been the subject of some debate. Some investigators claim a definite role for these studies as sensitive indicants, whereas others question whether the time and effort consumed in their performance offers any advantages above conventional clinical methods. Certainly the ability to provide more specific information in these rather common clinical settings would be of prime importance in arriving at medical decisions, but also of significant human value in dealing with the families of comatose patients. Clinical signs used to predict eventual outcome at times can be misleading—both unduly optimistic or pessimistic. Several investigators feel that evoked potentials offer significant help in such cases. For example, the situation where there is an intact BAER with absent somatosensory evoked response (SSER) has been, in certain hands, a reliable indicator of a chronic vegetative state in children who have sustained hypoxic cerebral injuries (Frank et al., 1985).

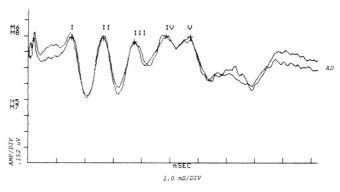

B

Figure 3-18. (A) Left-sided BAER has prolonged I–III interpeak interval and I–V interpeak is 0.48 msec longer than I–V on the right BAER. (B) Normal BAER, right ear. (C) CT scan demonstrating left cerebellopontine angle lesion thought to be epidermoid tumor (Case 13).

There are points that we would make that may differ from previous reports. First, it has been our experience that the performance of these studies, notably the BAER and SSER, are not without technical difficulty. The intensive care setting and the condition of comatose patients, those with serious head trauma who have undergone surgery, make these difficult patients from whom to obtain data. In general, the somatosensory evoked response has been considered a most useful indicator of outcome but, in particular, we find that this procedure is difficult to perform and in some cases impossible. We feel that its absence should be interpreted with caution, and abnormalities can be present unrelated to the issue at hand (e.g., underlying cervical spondylitis). With regard the BAER, the matter of pre-existent auditory pathology or temporal bone fracture limits the index of certitude. In the intensive care unit (ICU), the high gains and high-intensity input levels used often create added technical difficulties.

As would be expected, absent BAERs and SSERs are strongly associated with unfavorable outcome (death). We found that the elapsed time following the initial insult, whatever the cause, and the measurement of the BAER is an important factor. Our experience is that responses obtained after a significant lapse following the insult may show total absence of all wave forms, including wave I. Although in a pure sense, when no waves are seen little can be said whether the dysfunction is central or secondary to lack of sensory input. We feel, however, that bilateral loss of all wave forms is a grave prognostic sign and more likely associated with autolysis of the organ of Corti and cellular loss of the cochlear nucleus than with pre-existent hearing impairment (Kaga et al., 1985) (Fig. 3-19). Although absence of all waves beyond I and II has generally been associated with cerebral death, a report in a 33-month-old child (following near drowning) who was treated with barbituate coma, demonstrated serial brainstem responses that totally disappeared and subsequently reappeared (Taylor et al., 1983). This was attributed to transient middle ear dysfunction but indeed the implications of this observation are sobering and reemphasize the need for clinical correlation and cautious interpretation. Beyond this isolated case report, we have found several MS patients with only moderate clinical involvement who have preservation of solely waves I and II (see discussion of Case 9). We feel that these situations regarding the BAER point up a level of uncertainty that hinders its value in cerebral death determination.

It has long been realized that the BAER is more resistant to alteration, in patients comatose for a variety of reasons, than are the clinical brainstem reflexes such as the oculocephalic or oculovestibular reflexes. It is our opinion that conclusions should not be based on the results of one isolated BAER; particularly, a BAER that falls within normal range should not be used to predict a favorable clinical outcome. Serial measures and persistent trends, in conjunction with improving clinical signs, are more reliable. It is common in our experience to see a relatively normal BAER associated with absent oculovestibular and oculocephalic reflexes followed shortly by deterioration and ultimate cerebral death (see discussion Case 17). In summary, we find a very limited role for the BAER in the determination of brain death. We also have found that prognostication in comatose patients remains a difficult enterprise. We acknowledge that at times clinical determination can be unduly pessimistic but perceive that multimodality evoked potentials, including both the BAER and SSER, have difficulties in their administration and interpretation. Although totally absent responses or a response with preservation only of wave I or II consistently indicates a poor prognosis (death), an isolated normal response does not ensure a good clinical result, and only serial measures and their relationship to the neurologic exam and overall medical status are relevant. In light of our experience and the discrepancies in published findings, we seriously question the routine use of these studies in clinical practice from both a medical and cost-effective basis. On the other hand, we agree that there are significant gaps in our ability to provide prognostic information in the comatose individual, and the continuation of valid research in this application of evoked potentials is warranted. In Chapter 5, Dr. James Hall has presented a more favorable experience with evoked potentials in cerebral trauma.

CEREBRAL DEATH

Case 14

This patient was a 30-year-old female who ingested a massive dose of tricyclic antidepressants. Respirations were agonal after resuscitation (CPR) and all brainstem reflexes were absent. The EEG was isoelectric. BAERs (Fig. 3-19 A & B) showed absence of all waves, including wave I. After 36 hours, the tricyclic level was zero and artificial support devices were discontinued.

In light of the fact that there was no wave I, a specific comment regarding brain death could not be made. Without wave I, the integrity of the auditory end-organ mechanism is not assured. Despite this, it is a common situation to find absence of all waves in cerebral death (77 percent of cases; Goldie et al., 1981). This could be related to autolysis of the organ of Corti and cochlear nucleus (Fig. 3-19 C & D) rather than predicated on any pre-existent hearing loss. The usual resistance to change of the BAERs to drug intoxication was absent and tends to support irreversible CNS dysfunction. The ability to demonstrate sequential dropout of waves and, ultimately, wave I dropout requires the fortuitous timing of repeated trials. In our opinion, the clinical impact of this information rarely justifies the effort.

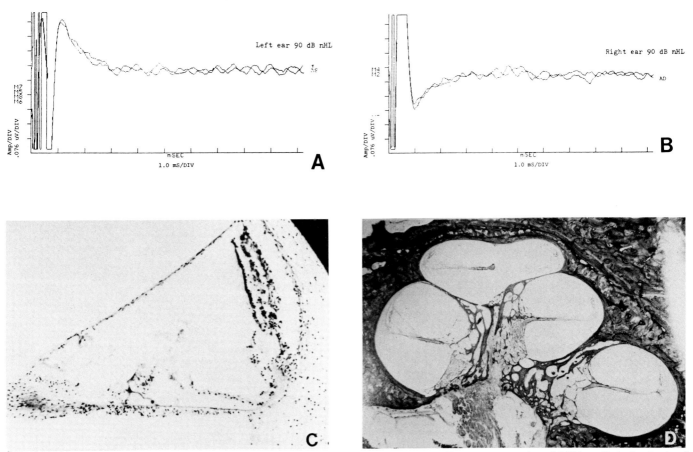

Figure 3-19. (A & B) BAER from both left (a) and right (b) ear show total absence of all waves in a patient fulfilling clinical criteria of cerebral death. (C & D) This demonstrates the cochlear abnormalities on postmortem examination, performed 3 hours after death, of an individual who demonstrated gradual disruption of the BAER and ultimately loss of all waves including wave I. There was almost complete loss of the organ of Corti (d), profound separation of the tectorial membrane from the hair cells, and disintegration of Reissner's membrane (c). These changes are felt to have occurred during the comatose period and are not related to postmortem autolysis. It should be considered that autolysis of the organ of Corti and disruption of the cochlear nucleus may be responsible for totally absent BAERs in the comatose state (Case 14). From Kaga, K, & Takamori, A, & Mizutani, T, et al., 1985. Auditory pathology of brain death. *Ann Neurol, 18,* p. 362. With permission.

PROLONGED COMA FOLLOWING CEREBRAL TRAUMA

Case 15

This 28-year-old woman was found in a field by her family when she failed to return home from horseback riding. She was comatose and responded to noxious stimuli with bilateral decerebrate responses. Oculocephalic and cold water calorics were initially absent. BAERs were preserved (Figure 3-20 A,B). CT scan demonstrated bifrontal contusional hemorrhages (Figure 3-20 E & F). Spontaneous respirations persisted. Early in her hospital course, she exhibited

profound lability in blood pressure, pulse, and temperature. Her family was presented with a poor prognostic picture.

She remained comatose for 2 weeks, with bilateral decerebrate responses. Thereafter, gradual slow improvement began and after 1 month she was transferred to a rehabilitation hospital. Since that time, persistent progress has continued and she has returned home with an overall excellent recovery.

This case demonstrates a not infrequent situation in which BAERs are preserved despite absent clinical brainstem reflexes. Of note is the improvement in both morphology and latency values of the BAER with time (Figure 3-20 C,D). Obviously, normal BAERs indicate a better prognosis that do completely absent response or tracings with multiple absent waves, but an isolated normal BAER cannot reliably predict a good outcome.

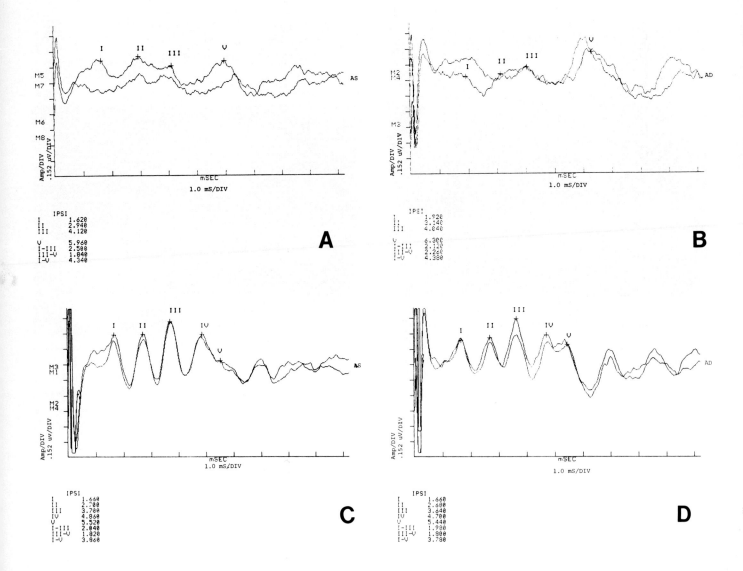

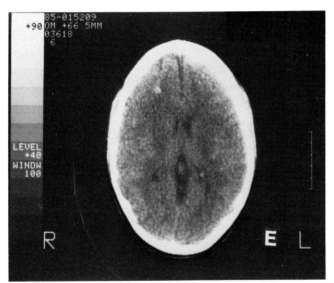
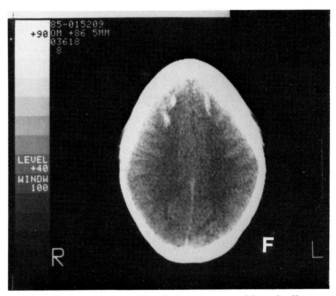

Figure 3-20. (A & B) BAERs obtained from patient in case #15 shortly after her head injury. Morphology is poor although all waves are preserved. (C & D) BAERs obtained 1 week later with improvement in morphology and reduction in absolute and interpeak latencies. (E & F) CT scan of brain obtained at time of admission with bilateral frontal contusional hemorrhage (Case 15).

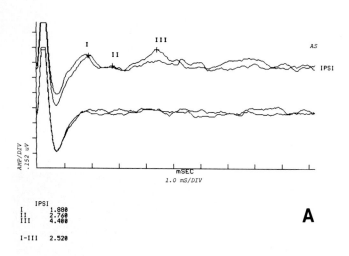

IPSI
I   1.880
II 2.760
III 4.400

I-III 2.520

A

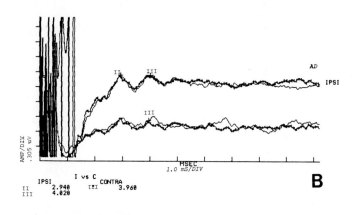

IPSI   I vs C   CONTRA
II 2.940   III 3.960
III 4.020

B

PONTINE HEMORRHAGE

Case 16

This 77-year-old white male was brought to an emergency room in coma. Several minutes prior to his change in mental status, he had complained of nausea and was unable to stand. CT demonstrates extensive pontine bleeding (Figure 3-21 C). Respirations remained irregular. Ice water calorics, oculocephalic reflexes, and pupillary reflexes were absent. Once he was removed from the respirator, the irregular respirations continued for 3 hours and he ultimately expired. BAERs (Figure 3-21 A & B) performed shortly before he was removed from the respirator show waves I and III and waves II and III, although an exact identification is far from certain. Complex technical factors frequently distort the results in the ICU. In the severely abnormal state, the BAER signal approaches that of the ambient noise, and in our experience this restricts its ability to definitively evaluate the cessation of brainstem function and cerebral death. In Figure 3-21 B a large stimulus artifact is demonstrated during the first millisecond. These data point up the problems in both technique and interpretation when the BAER is used in this setting.

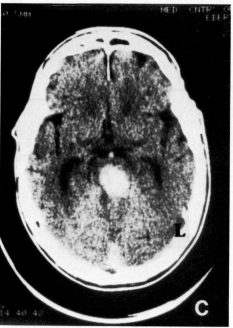

Figure 3-21. (A & B) BAER left ear (A) and right ear (B) in patient with pontine hemorrhage. (C) CT scan with extensive pontine hemorrhage (Case 16).

COMA FOLLOWING HYPOXIC-ISCHEMIC CEREBRAL INJURY

Case 17

This 79-year-old white female had a cardiopulmonary arrest several days after a hip replacement. Despite on-the-spot resuscitation, the patient immediately developed myoclonic seizures. Clinical brainstem reflexes, oculocephalic and oculovestibular, were absent. EEG, BAER, and SSER from the same day are presented in Figure 3-22 A–E. The BAERs and SSERs are remarkably normal. The following morning, the patient no longer exhibited spontaneous respirations. She became hypotensive and her clinical exam was consistent with cerebral death. The ventilator was discontinued at the request of the family. This case is presented to demonstrate that an isolated normal evoked response cannot be given undue significance and only serial observations over time should be used to prognosticate.

THE BAER IN PARENCHYMAL LESIONS OF THE BRAINSTEM

Each month, additional conditions associated with abnormalities in the BAER are reported. The scope of this diversity spans conditions as heterogeneous as migraine, Guillain-Barré syndrome, and Ondine's curse. Although these observations are interesting, there is nothing distinctive in the associations that would validate more widespread use of the BAER.

One area that we have found to be of consequence involves parenchymal lesions of the brainstem, using the BAER as a

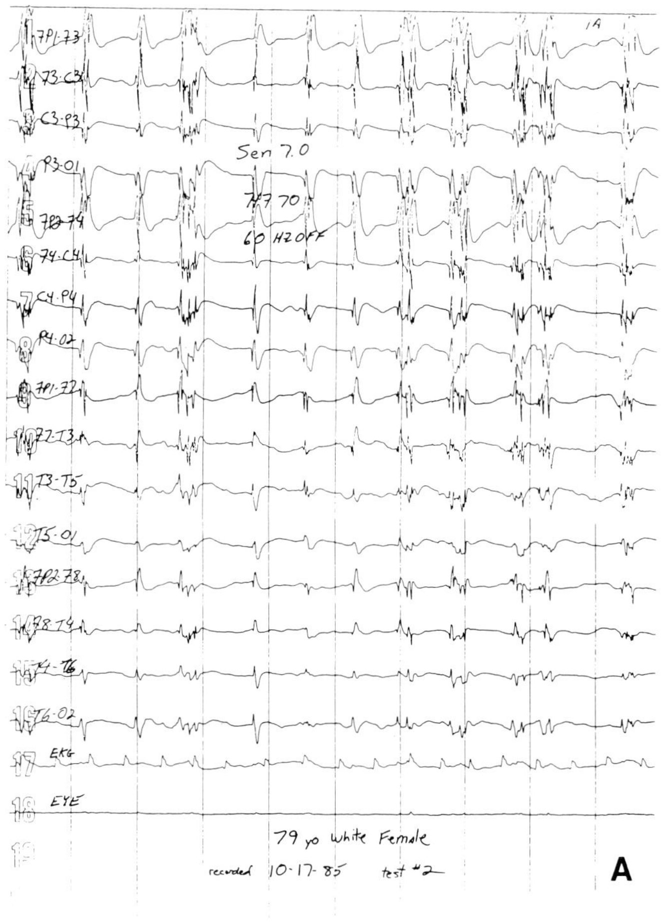

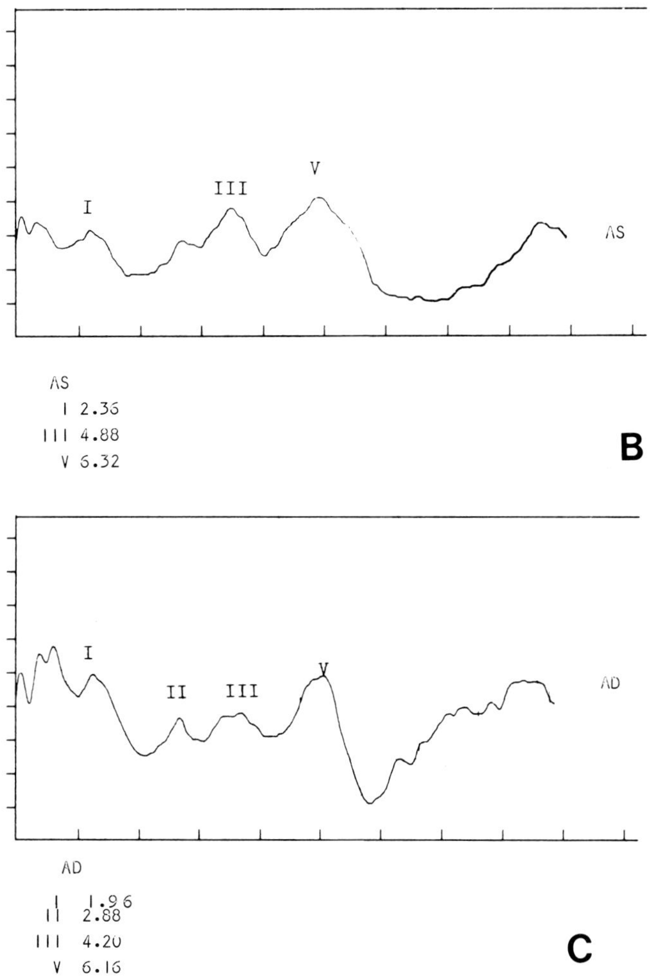

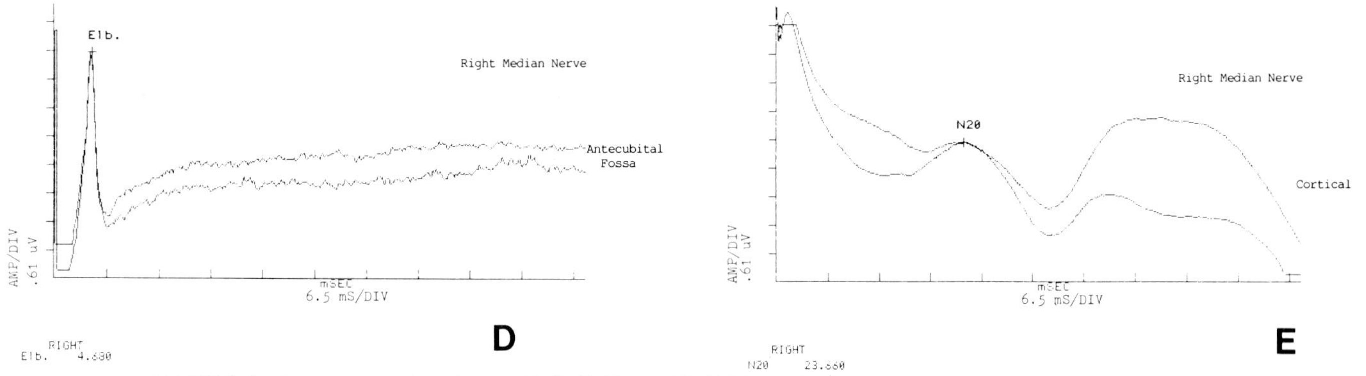

Figure 3-22. (A) EEG during postanoxic seizure. (B & C) Normal BAERs in this comatose individual. (E & F) Normal somatosensory evoked response using right median nerve stimulation (Case 17).

method of confirming abnormalities seen or not seen on radiologic studies (CT and MRI). In general, the evaluation of the brainstem tends to be its least sensitive region of resolution for CT. Early experience with MRI indicates that it offers a distinct improvement, but the specificity and significance of these "areas of increased signal" are not strictly defined. The BAER provides a different technologic probe to cross-check abnormalities suggested on clinical or radiologic grounds.

We present a variety of lesions, such as a brainstem stroke, a brainstem glioma, and a brainstem hamartoma, along with the CT and MRI scans. Once again, there is nothing characteristic in the BAER abnormalities specific for a particular lesion. Although interpeak intervals remain a preferred method of interpretation, there is frequently more extensive morphologic distortion of the BAER ipsilateral to the brainstem lesion. This

distortion takes the shape of attenuated or absent later waves, IV and V, but also wave III. As with demyelinating disease, intrinsic brainstem lesions can produce distortion of multiple waves but are generally not associated with pure-tone hearing loss. We have found multiple situations in which clinical findings and BAER abnormalities have existed in the face of a normal CT. MRI has clarified many of these discrepancies.

BRAINSTEM GLIOMA

Case 18

This 28-year-old male developed right-sided facial numbness, ataxia, a change in the tone of his voice, and increasing difficulty swallowing liquids. CT and MRI are demonstrated in Figure 3-23 C & D. Biopsy confirmed the diagnosis of brainstem glioma. BAERs are abnormal bilaterally with absence of multiple later wave components, particularly on the right. (Figure 3-23 A & B). Radiation therapy improved clinical symptoms but did not change the BAER.

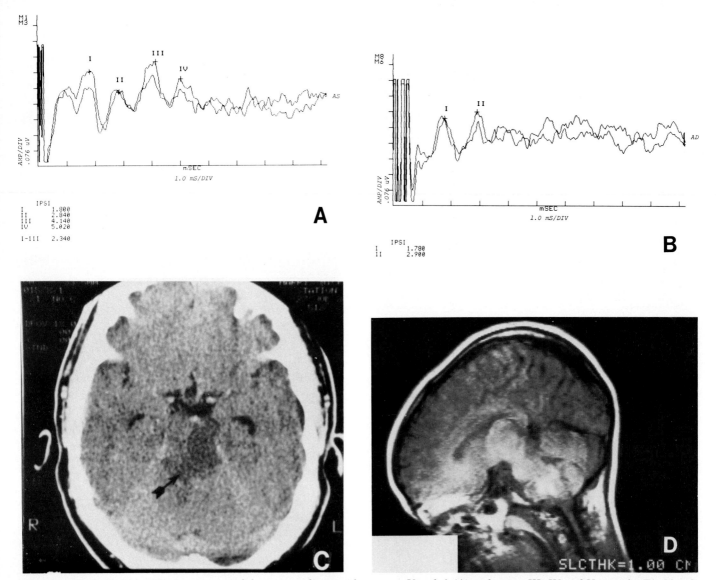

Figure 3-23. (A & B) BAERs in patient with brainstem glioma without wave V on left (A) and waves III, IV and V on right (B). Muscle artifact degrades the response. (C) CT demonstrates hypodense lesion of brainstem glioma. (D) MRI gives more detailed picture of extent of glioma. Arrow directed toward extensive area of increased signal in pons and mid brain (Case 18).

BRAINSTEM INFARCTION

Case 19

This 60-year-old male noted sudden onset of diplopia and ataxia in November of 1984. CT scan was normal. BAERs (Figure 3-24 A & B) were abnormal in that both the I–V and III–V interpeak intervals were prolonged on the right side. He did fairly well until April of 1985, when he became severely ataxic, and quadriparetic, and had difficulty dealing with copious secretions. Once again the CT scan was normal, but posterior fossa angiography revealed extensive atherosclerosis involving the vertebral-basilar system. MRI (Fig. 3-24 E & F) demonstrated multiple ares of increased signal within the brainstem, considered to be consistent with infarction. Repeat BAERs (Figure 3-24 C and D) in May of 1985 showed further degradation, with absent waves IV and V on the right and a change in the morphology on the left side with attenuation of waves IV and V. These changes were felt to be consistent with recurrent ischemic infarction within the brainstem parenchyma. The clinical findings as well as the BAER both favored predominantly right-sided brainstem involvement. We have found the BAER to be sensitive to brainstem infarction in cases where CT is normal and MRI equivocal. As previously mentioned, however, there is nothing specific in the abnormalities particular for vascular disease.

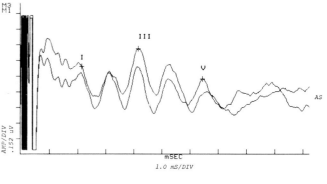

A

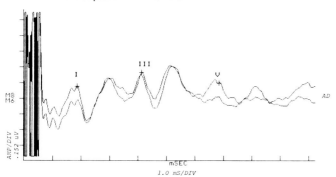

B

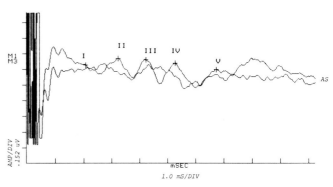

C

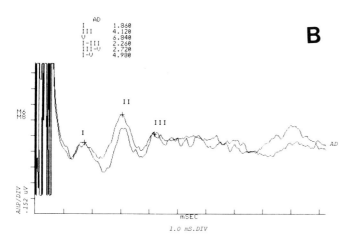

D

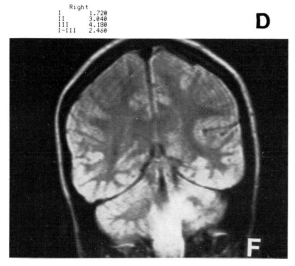

F

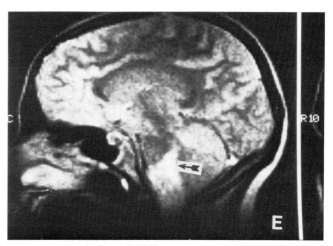

E

Figure 3-24. (A & B) BAERs in patient following episode of suspected brainstem infarction. Right side (B) is abnormal with prolongation of I–III and I–V interpeaks. (C & D) BAER in same individual 6 months later and following another episode of brainstem ischemia are bilaterally abnormal with extensive disruption on the right (D). (E & F) MRI, sagittal (E) and coronal (F) views, demonstrating the abnormality particularly in the right brainstem parenchyma (Case 19).

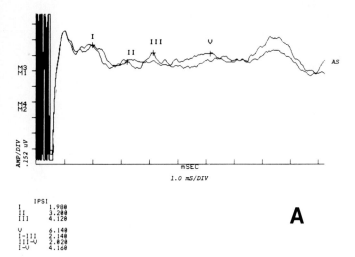

IPSI

I	1.980
II	3.200
III	4.120
V	6.140
I–III	2.140
III–V	2.020
I–V	4.160

A

BRAINSTEM TUMOR

Case 20

This 18-year-old male experienced one year of increasing hiccoughs. Over a 27-month period, his voice became very hoarse and he had difficulty with copious secretions. CT (Figure 3-25 C) demonstrated an isolated area of calcification in the middle cerebellar peduncle near the dentate nucleus. MRI and BAERs are demonstrated in Figure 3-25 A,B,D,E. Biopsy of this lesion led to its diagnosis as a hamartoma. BAERs from the right ear (Figure 3-25 B) show normal morphology and latencies. On the left side (Fig. 3-25 A), however, all waves beyond wave I are severely attenuated. MRI (Fig. 3-25 D,E) is clearly more effective than is the CT demonstrating the extent of the involvement into the parenchyma of the pons. Although hearing loss on the left side was minimal, profound degradation of the morphology of the BAER is evident. Rather than subtle differences in interpeak latencies, we have found these more drastic morphologic changes to be a common occurrence with intrinsic lesions of the brainstem.

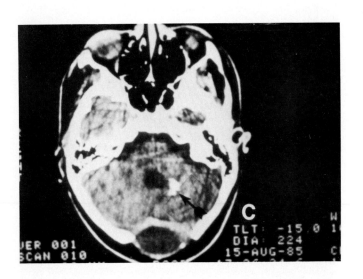

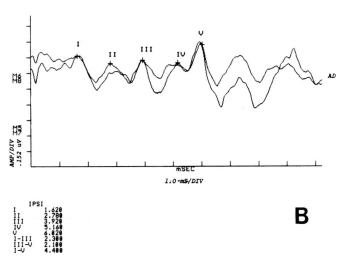

IPSI

I	1.620
II	2.780
III	3.920
IV	5.160
V	6.020
I–III	2.300
III–V	2.100
I–V	4.400

B

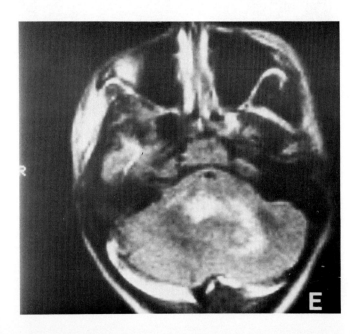

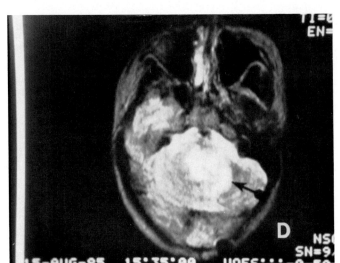

Figure 3-25. (A) Abnormal left BAER with severe attenuation of later waves III, IV & V. (B) Normal right BAER. (C) CT scan of calcific lesion in left cerebellar hemisphere. (D & E) MRI scans more clearly indicate tumor (hamartoma) in left cerebellar hemisphere and pons (Case 20).

CEREBELLAR TUMOR INVADING THE BRAINSTEM

Case 21

This 62-year-old female presented with a 3-month history of vague lightheadedness and unsteadiness walking. Audiogram and ENG were normal and the BAER demonstrated in Figure 3-26 A and B shows excellent morphology and normal latencies. MRI (Fig. 3-26 C & D) demonstrates a large left cerebellar lesion with compression of both the fourth ventricle and brainstem with obliteration of the prepontine cistern on the right side. Increased signal intensity was identified in both of the cerebellar hemispheres as well as the left middle cerebellar peduncle and dorsal brainstem. Surgery confirmed an astrocytoma. The BAER (Fig. 3-26 A & B) is normal bilaterally. This underscores the need for educating referring physicians regarding the fact that a normal BAER does not imply a normal brainstem, but, rather, implies that the peripheral and central auditory tracts are not involved.

CONCLUSION

The preceding discussion was but one perspective regarding the utility of the BAER. A concerted attempt was made to differentiate between clinical research and clinical practice, and to emphasize that the former should precede the latter. Although abnormalities in the BAER have been described in a variety of diverse neurologic conditions, it is our opinion that its application in clinical practice remains quite limited. Despite these limitations, the test can yield important information and be complementary to other modes of neurodiagnosis. We would regard the current state of the BAER, as well as the other modalities of evoked potentials, as an important preliminary step in expanding and objectifying the physiologic aspects of the clinical neurologic examination.

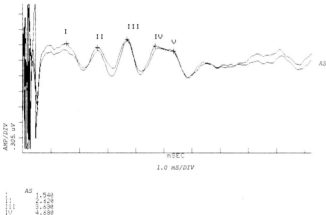
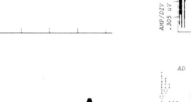
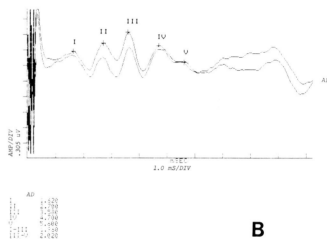
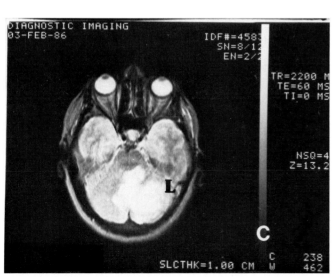
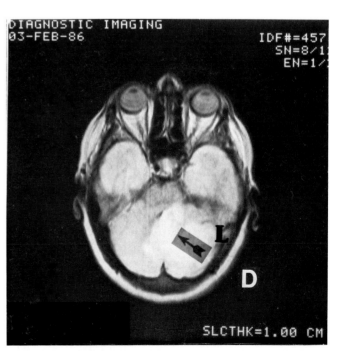

Figure 3-26. (A & B) Normal BAERs bilaterally. (C & D) MRI demonstrates large left cerebellar astrocytoma (Case 21).

ACKNOWLEDGMENTS

The author is extremely appreciative of the technical assistance provided by Shelle Shimon, M.S., Jean Taylor, R.N., and DeeAnn Wilson. He is also thankful for the generous input on acoustic neuromas furnished by Charles M. Luetje, M.D., of Kansas City, Missouri.

REFERENCES

Aminoff, M, Davis, S, & Panitch, H (1984). Serial evoked potential studies in patients with definite multiple sclerosis. *Arch Neurol, 41*, 1197–1202

Chiappa, K, Harrison, J, Brooks, E, & Young, R (1980). Brainstem auditory evoked responses in 200 patients with multiple sclerosis. *Ann Neurol, 7*, 135–143

Chiappa, K & Yiannikas, C (1983). Evoked potentials in clinical medicine. Brainstem auditory evoked potentials: Methodology (105–143). Brainstem auditory evoked potentials: Interpretation (144–190). New York: Raven Press

Davis, S, Aminoff, M, & Berg, B (1985). Brainstem auditory evoked potentials in children with brainstem or cerebellar dysfunction. *Arch Neurol, 42*, 156–160

Eggermont, JJ, & Don, M (1986). Mechanisms of central conduction time prolongation in brainstem auditory evoked potentials. *Arch Neurol, 43*, 116–120

Eisen, A, Paty, DE, & Hoirch, M (1982). Altered supernormality in multiple sclerosis peripheral nerve. *Muscle Nerve 4*, 411–414

Frank, L, Furgiuele, T, & Etheridge, J (1985). Prediction of chronic vegetative state in children using evoked potentials. *Neurology, 35*, 931–934

Fria, T (1980). The auditory brainstem response: Background and clinical applications in: Schwartz, D.M. & Bess, F.H. (eds). Monographs in contemporary audiology. Minnesota: Maico Hearing Instruments 2 (2) 1:38

Goldie, W, Chiappa, K, Young, R, & Brooks, E (1981). Brainstem auditory and short-latency somatosensory evoked responses in brain death. *Neurology (NY), 31*, 248–256

Hecox, K (1983). Brainstem auditory evoked responses: Technical factors, Part I. *Nicolet Potentials, Vol 2, 1*, 19–24

Kaga, K, Takamori, A, Mizutani, T, Nagai, T, & Marsh, RR (1985). The auditory pathology of brain death as revealed by auditory evoked potentials. *Ann Neurology*, Sept: 18(3), 360–364

Moller, AR, & Jannetta, PJ (1983). Auditory evoked potentials recorded from the cochlear nucleus and its vicinity in man. *J Neurosurg, 59, 1013–1018, 1983*

Norton, W (1981). Biochemistry of myelin (93–114). Waxman, S: Clinicopathological correlations in multiple sclerosis and related diseases (169–180). In, Advances in Neurology, Vol. 31 New York: Raven Press

Regan, D (1981). Psychophysical tests of vision and hearing in patients with multiple sclerosis (217–235). In, Advances in Neurology, Vol. 31. New York: Raven Press

Sekiya, T, Iwabuchi, T, Kamata, S, & Ishida, T (1985). Deterioration of auditory evoked potentials during cerebellopontine angle manipulations. *J Neurosurg 63*, 598–607

Smith, CG: (1981). Serial Dissection Of The Human Brain, page 60. Urban & Schwarzenberg. Baltimore-Munich

Taylor, M, Houston, B, Lowry, N (1983). Recovery of auditory brainstem responses after a severe hypoxic ischemic insult. *New England J Med*, Vol 309, 1169–1170

BIBLIOGRAPHY

Anderson, D, Bundlie, S, & Rockswold, G (1984). Multimodality evoked potentials in closed head trauma. *Arch Neurol, 41*, 369–374

Chiappa, K, & Young, R (1985). Evoked responses. Overused, underused, or misused? *Arch Neurol, 42*, 76–77

Daniels, DL, Herfkins, R, Koehler, PR, Millen, SJ, Shaffer, KA, Williams, AL, Haughton, VM (1984). Magnetic resonance imaging of the internal auditory canal. *Radiology, 151*(1) 105–108

Davis, R, & Cunningham, P (1984). Prognostic factors in severe injury. *Surg Gynecol Obstet, 159*, 597–604

DeWeese, D, & Saunders, W (1982). Textbook of otolaryngology. Hearing Losses (347–373). St. Louis: The C.V. Mosby Company

Eisen, A (1983). Neurophysiology in multiple sclerosis, 615–629. In, Neurologic clinics, multiple sclerosis, neurology clinics, Vol. I, 3. Philadelphia: W.B. Saunders Co

Garg, B, Markand, O, & Bustion, P (1982). Brainstem auditory evoked responses in hereditary motorsensory neuropathy: Site of origin of wave II. *Neurology, 32*, 1017–1019

Graham, M, & Sataloff, R (1984). Acoustic tumors in the young adult. *Arch Otolaryngol* Vol 110, 405–407

Greenberg, R, & Ducker, T (1982). Evoked potentials in the clinicl neurosciences. *J Neurosurg, 56*, 1–18

Hall, J, Brown, D, & Mackey-Hargadine, J (1985). Pediatric applications of serial auditory brainstem and middle-latency evoked response recordings. *Int J Pediatric Otorhinolaryngology 9*, 201–218

Hall, J, Mackey-Hargadine, J, & Kim, E (1985). Auditory brainstem response in determination of brain death. *Arch Otolaryngology, 3*, 613–620

Hammond, E, Wilder, J, Goodman, I, Hunter, S (1985). Auditory brainstem potentials with unilateral pontine hemorrhage. *Arch Neurol 42*, 767–768

Harner, S, & Laws, E (1983). Clinical findings in patients with acoustic neurinoma. *Mayo Clin Proc, 58*, 721–728

Hecox, K, Cone, B, & Blaw, M (1981). Brainstem auditory evoked response in the diagnosis of pediatric neurologic diseases. *Neurology, 31*, 832–845

Hecox, K (1984). Brainstem auditory evoked response: Audiologic applications, Part II. *Nicolet Potentials, 39*, 41–47

Hopf, H, & Eysholdt, M (1978). Impaired refractory periods of peripheral sensory nerves in multiple sclerosis. *Ann Neurol, 4*, 499–501

Karnaze, D, Weiner, J, & Marshall, L (1985). Auditory evoked potentials in coma after closed head injury: A clinical-neurophysiologic coma scale for predicting outcome. *Neurology, 35*, 1122–1126

Karnaze, D, Marshall, L, McCarthy, C, Klauber, M, & Bickford, R (1982). Localizing and prognostic value of auditory evoked responses in coma after closed head injury. *Neurology, 32*, 299–302

Kimura, J (1985). Abuse and misuse of evoked potentials as a diagnostic test. *Arch Neurol, 42*, 78–80

Levine, R, & Montgomery, W (1984). Monitoring auditory evoked potentials during acoustic neuroma surgery. Insights into the mechanism of the hearing loss. *Ann Otol Rhinol Laryngol, 93*, 116–123

Lindsay, K, Carlin, J, Kennedy, I, Fry, J, McInnes, A, & Teasdale, GM (1981). Evoked potentials in severe head injury-analysis and relation to outcome. *J Neurol, Neurosurg and Psychiatry, 44*, 796–802

Long, K, & Allen, N (1984). Brainstem auditory evoked potentials following Ondine's curse. *Arch Neurol, 41*, 1109–1110

Luetje, C, & Whittaker, C (1980). Acoustic tumors. *JKMS, 81-7*, 343–347

Newlon, P, & Greenberg, R (1984). Evoked potentials in severe head injury. *J Trauma, 24*, 1, 61–65

Ochs, R, Markand, O, & DeMyer, W (1979). Brainstem auditory evoked responses in leukodystrophies. *Neurology, 29*, 1089–1093

Owen, J, & Davis, H (1985). Evoked potential testing, clinical applications. 55–108. Brainstem auditory evoked responses. Orlando, FL: Grune & Stratton.

Recommended standards for the clinical practice of evoked potentials. *J Clin Neurophysiol, 1*, 6–53, 1984

Rosenberg, C, Wogensen, K, & Starr, A (1984). Auditory brainstem and middle and long latency evoked potentials in coma. *Arch Neurol, 41*, 835–838

Schiff, J, Cracco, R, & Cracco, J (1985). Brainstem auditory evoked potentials in Guillain-Barré syndrome. *Neurology, 35*, 771–773

Stockard, J, & Rossiter, V (1977). Clinical and pathologic correlates of brainstem auditory response abnormalities. *Neurology, 27*, 316–325

Stockard, J, Stockard, JE, & Sharbrough, F (1977). Detection and localization of occult lesions with brainstem auditory responses. *Mayo Clin Proc, 52*, 761–769

Strickbine-Van Reet, P, Glaze, D, & Hrachovy, R (1984). A preliminary prospective neurophysiological study of coma in children. *AJDC, 138*, 492–495

Tsubokawa, T, Nishimoto, H, Yamamoto, T, Kitamura, M, Katayama, Y, & Moriyasu, N (1980). Assessment of brainstem damage by the auditory brainstem response in acute severe head injury. *J Neurol Neurosurg Psychiatry, 43,* 1005–1011

Verma, N, & Lynn, G (1985). Auditory evoked responses in multiple sclerosis. *Arch Otolaryngol, 111,* 22–44

Williams, J, Gomes, F, Drudge, O, & Kessler, M (1985). Predicting outcome from closed head injury by early assessment of trauma severity. *J Neurosurg, 61,* 581–585

Louise D. Resor

4

The Brainstem Auditory Evoked Response in Pediatric Neurologic Practice

The brainstem auditory evoked response (BAER) is a series of far-field potentials originating from the tracts and nuclei of the auditory system.

The response consists of a series of waves labeled I through V. The presumed generators of the response includes the eighth nerve, the cochlear nucleus, the superior olive, and the lateral lemniscus and inferior colliculus. In clinical neurologic practice, it is abnormalities of interpeak latency, waveform, and morphology that are of particular interest. In general, a I–III interpeak latency abnormality suggests a problem between the cochlea and the lower pons; a III–V interpeak latency abnormality suggests a disturbance between the lower pons and midbrain; and a I–V interpeak latency abnormality suggests diffuse problems. However, there is no BAER abnormality that is specific for a particular neurologic disease.

The principles of recording and interpreting BAEPs have been discussed elsewhere. It is the purpose of this chapter to review the applications of this technique in pediatric neurologic practice and to focus in particular on those clinical situations where BAERs provide information not accessible by other diagnostic techniques.

BRAINSTEM AUDITORY EVOKED POTENTIALS: MATURATION AND NORMS

Brainstem auditory evoked potentials can be recorded in the premature infant as young as 28–30 weeks (Starr et al., 1977; Despland and Galambos, 1980, 1982). Some authors have noted that BAERs are frequently not elicited in "normal" infants of 30–34 weeks gestation, but if stimuli of sufficient intensity (90–110 dB) are used, BAERs can be recorded with regularity after 30 weeks (Roberts et al., 1982; Bradford et al., 1985). The absolute threshold for eliciting BAERs reaches 20 dB by about 5 months of age (Hecox and Burkard, 1982).

In adult patients, age has little impact on interpeak latencies and waveform. However, age is extremely important when determining interpeak latencies and BAER morphology in preterm infants as well as in children under 1 year. In the normal premature infant, BAERs often consist of 3 components: waves I, III, and V. Compared to adult norms, these components shorten significantly in latency, increase in amplitude, and appear at lower intensities with the approach of term (Fig. 4-1) (Despland and Galambos, 1982).

The maturational changes in BAER waveform and interpeak latency that conventionally occur with age have been well described in the literature (Salamy and McKean, 1976; Mochizuki et al., 1982). Waves I, III, and V can routinely be seen in the premature and term infant, while wave II appears to differentiate clearly at about 4–6 weeks. By 3–6 months, the characteristic BAER morphology emerges (Fig. 4-2). The amplitude of wave V increases to achieve an adult value at about 2–3 years of age. It increases further during years four and five before achieving an adult value (Fig. 4-3).

While peripheral auditory transmission time (wave I latency) approaches an adult value from the first months of life, the maturation of central transmission (I–V interpeak latency) proceeds more slowly. There appears to be an abrupt decrease in central transmission time between birth and 6 weeks, with an-

Clinical Atlas of Auditory Evoked Potentials
ISBN 0-8089-1896-6

28 week gestation female

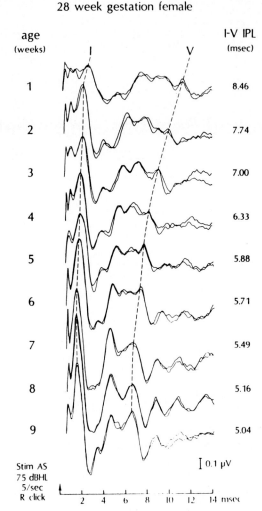

Figure 4-1. Serial studies of normal 28-week-gestation infant. Over the 9-week period of study, wave I decreased by 1.36 msec and wave V by 4.78 msec. The I–V interpeak latency (IPL) decreased in a non-linear fashion, with greater weekly changes occurring in early prematurity (> 0.7 msec/week). Note that the latencies are far more stable over time as term is approached. Component identification was confirmed by simultaneous recording of vertex to contralateral ear. From Stockard, JE, & Westmoreland, BF (1981). Technical considerations in the recording and interpretation of the brainstem auditory evoked potential for neonatal neurologic diagnosis. *Technology, 21*:31–54. With permission.

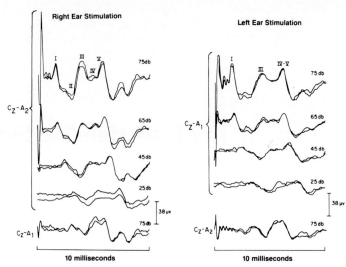

Figure 4-2. BAERs in a normal 2-month-old.

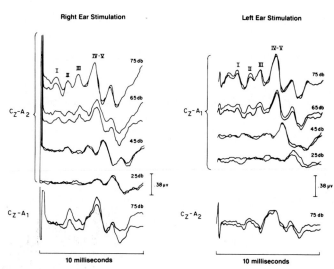

Figure 4-3. Normal BAERs in a normal 3-year-old.

other significant drop occurring between 6 months and 1 year. By 12–18 months, central transmission time is essentially that of an adult (Salamy and McKean, 1976; Mochizuki et al., 1982). (Table 4-1).

TECHNICAL FACTORS INVOLVED IN RECORDING AND INTERPRETING BAERs IN NEONATES AND YOUNG CHILDREN

The technical factors involved in the measurement and interpretation of neonatal BAERs have been described by Stockard and Westmoreland (1981). Several features are of particular note. Pressure on the outer ear in the newborn and pre-term infant can collapse the compliant canal wall. Consequently, the stimulating earphone should be hand-held over the test ear and the contralateral earphone embedded in a soft mattress. When wave I is prolonged in the neonate, canal collapse should be considered.

Because of the potential for muscle contamination and the general lower response amplitude, testing should be done while the infant is in the sleep state. In the newborn, this is routinely accomplished after the infant has been fed and swaddled. In older babies and uncooperative children, thirty to fifty mg/kg of chloral hydrate (P.O.) usually provides adequate sedation.

For infants and young children, as well as older youngsters unable to cooperate for click threshold determination by ques-

Table 4-1 Mean and Standard Deviation of Peak Latency (in msec) in
Different Age Groups

		Number	Waves	I	III	V	I–V
Newborn							
	Mochizuki et al. (1982)	14	Mean	1.58	4.35	6.76	5.18
			SD	.13	.19	.25	.26
	Salamy & McKean (1976)	90	Mean	2.12	4.89	7.06	5.12
			SD	.35	.35	.38	.29
3 months							
	Mochizuki et al. (1982)	21	Mean	1.49	4.12	6.46	4.96
			SD	.12	.14	.23	.20
	Salamy & McKean (1976)	23	Mean	1.82	4.15	6.40	4.67
			SD	.27	.20	.29	.35
6 months							
	Mochizuki et al. (1982)	17	Mean	1.49	4.05	6.37	4.87
			SD	.09	.18	.20	.18
	Salamy & McKean (1976)	14	Mean	1.74	4.16	6.34	4.63
			SD	.02	.32	.32	.30
1 year							
	Mochizuki et al. (1982)	18	Mean	1.47	3.88	6.06	4.58
			SD	.09	.13	.26	.24
	Salamy & McKean (1976)	10	Mean	1.71	3.92	5.93	4.20
			SD	.21	.25	.30	.36

tioning, click intensity of 75–85 dB HL can be used. In the pre-verbal and uncooperative patient, even those referred purely for brainstem evaluation, threshold testing is advisable.

BAERs IN THE NEONATAL INTENSIVE CARE UNIT

BAERs can provide objective electrophysiologic assessment of auditory function in uncooperative, sleeping, and comatose patients. Consequently, BAERs have been advocated as a valuable hearing screen in the neonatal intensive care unit (ICU), where the incidence of significant hearing impairment is estimated to be as high as 8–20 percent. Despland and Galambos (1982) studied 100 patients in a neonatal intensive care unit, noting 14 patients with abnormal BAERs. One-half of these patients had significant hearing loss at follow-up, but transient BAER abnormalities are particularly common in this age group. Wave I prolongation and moderate threshold elevation, for example, are noted in a significant proportion of small pre-term infants. Several authors have pointed out that this pattern carries little prognostic significance in the pre-term infant (Roberts et al., 1982; Stockard et al., 1983; Stein et al., 1983). Threshold testing by BAERs should be done as close to term as possible, with follow-up 1 month post-term to avoid giving pathological significance to results reflective only of incomplete maturation.

Infants with persistent moderate threshold elevation and prolongation of Wave I latency, on the other hand, have a significant incidence of conductive hearing loss. Chronic otitis media is seen in 50–60 percent of infants in this group (Stockard et al., 1983). Persistent absence or a marked degree of wave I threshold elevation is associated with a significant incidence of sensorineural hearing impairment. Complete BAER absence (including wave I) to 110 dB stimulation appears, even in the small pre-term infant, seems to have a good correlation with subsequent hearing dysfunction. Bradford et al. (1985) studied BAERs in 117 newborns born at less than 33 weeks gestation. BAERs to 110 dB stimulation were absent in 10 infants studied after 30 weeks of age gestation. By 1 year of age, 9 out of 10 of these infants with absent BAERs in the neonatal period were shown to have sensorineural hearing loss that required hearing aids.

Persistent absence of BAERs has also been recorded in infants with clinical evidence of brainstem dysfunction with apparently normal hearing (Stockard et al., 1983). In infants with brainstem abnormalities, the BAER threshold may not be a reliable indicator of auditory sensitivity (Stockard and Westmoreland, 1981). This re-emphasizes the importance of maintaining an alertness to both audiologic and neurologic issues when interpreting results. In addition, the BAER as a measure of central auditory transmission has been used in the neonatal intensive care unit in assessing the integrity of brainstem structures particularly vulnerable to the usual perinatal stresses such as asphyxia and hyperbilirubinemia. As with peripheral conduction, central patterns of BAER abnormality, such as increased interpeak latencies, are also seen transiently in the small pre-term infant and appear to be of little prognostic significance (Stockard et al., 1983).

Hecox and Cone (1981) studied asphyxiated full-term infants and noted that markedly abnormal amplitude ratios, where wave I amplitude exceeded wave V amplitude, correlated with grossly abnormal neurological outcomes. Of 21 full-term infants in their study with grossly abnormal amplitude ratios, on follow-up, 15 had severe spastic quadriparesis and cognitive impairment and 6 were dead. On the other hand, these authors noted that normal amplitude ratios did not ensure a favorable neurological outcome; another 10 patients in their study with normal amplitude ratios were similarly severely neurologically impaired. Clearly, amplitude ratios are among the most variable BAER parameters and among the most susceptible to contamination by artifact and technical factors. It is recommended that amplitudes vary 20 percent or less in repeated trials to be considered prognostically significant. Stockard et al. (1983) noted that absence of later BAER components with preservation of wave I or severe V:I amplitude ratio reduction had a high correlation with neurologic impairment in follow-up. They also reported, however, the case of a premature child with only minimal sequelae of a perinatal hypoxic event despite having no recordable wave V from birth through the age of 8 months. Transient central BAER abnormalities can be seen in asphyxiated pre-term infants and are not incompatible with subsequent normal neurologic outcome (Stockard et al., 1983; Stein et al., 1983).

In the perinatal intensive care unit, BAERs would appear to have value both as an objective screen of auditory function as well as a measure of brainstem integrity. The transient nature of both central and peripheral BAER abnormalities in the pre-term and newborn infant suggests that the tests may have increased prognostic value when performed after a period of clinical stabilization. Follow-up BAER testing 1 month post-term in conjunction with further audiologic and neurologic assessments is important before any inferences can be made about ultimate hearing and neurodevelopmental outcome (Case 1, Fig. 4-4).

BAERs AND THE SUDDEN INFANT DEATH SYNDROME

Earlier reports noting the routine presence of central BAER abnormalities in patients with the near-miss sudden infant death syndrome (NMSIDS) suggested that BAERs could be used to detect at-risk infants (Nodar et al., 1980B; Orlowski et al., 1979). Several subsequent studies, however, have not shown a predictive value of BAERs in this setting (Gupta et al., 1981; Luders et al., 1984; Stockard, 1982). Luders et al., for example, studied 16 NMSIDS patients but noted only 1 patient with an interpeak latency outside the tolerance limit defined as normal. The marked discrepancy between these and the earlier studies may be due to a less stringent definition of BAER abnormality in the earlier studies. Stockard, in his longitudinal study of BAERs in NMSIDS patients, noted that while NMSIDS survi-

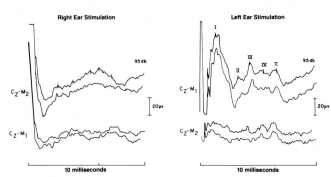

Figure 4-4. Case 1. BAERS in an 8-week-old infant. This infant was born at 37 weeks gestation. An emergency Cesarean section was performed for fetal distress, and cardiopulmonary resuscitation was required in the delivery room. The perinatal course was complicated by severe respiratory distress, hyperbilirubinemia and sepsis. The BAERs performed at 8 weeks show a markedly abnormal V–I amplitude ratio to left ear stimulation with no response obtainable below 80 dB. No BAER could be recorded to right ear stimulation. The youngster remains severely handicapped at 7 months of age with a spastic quadriparesis. The markedly abnormal V–I amplitude ratio to left ear stimulation correlated in this asphyxiated term infant with an abnormal neurological outcome. Serial testing in conjunction with further clinical assessment is preferred before making statements to anxiety-ridden parents about ultimate outcome.

vors have normal BAERs when compared as individuals to age-matched controls, most had mean I–V latency values 1–2.2 standard deviations greater than normal values. The degree of deviation from the mean in these patients appeared to correlate with the frequency and severity of apneic episodes, and was similar to that seen in babies with chronic hypoxemia due to congenital heart disease or chronic respiratory insufficiency. The only patient in this series to die from an apparent SIDS episode had normal central auditory conduction prior to several NMSIDS episodes.

The minimal BAER deviations seen in near-miss SIDS patients suggests that these deviations are secondary to repeated hypoxic events rather than reflective of a pre-existing brainstem abnormality causing apnea. At the present time, it would seem that BAERs have no predictive value in identifying infants at risk for the sudden infant death syndrome.

BAER IN MENINGITIS

Partial or total deafness continues to be a frequent and unpredictable complication of bacterial meningitis in childhood, despite advances in antibiotic therapy. Early estimates of the incidence of sensorineural hearing loss following meningitis were in the range of 3–5 percent (Swartz and Dodge, 1965). These earlier studies necessarily depended on conventional audiometry in the evaluation of hearing and contained a disproportionately small number of infants and very young children.

BAERs, on the other hand, provide an objective measure of auditory function as well as of brainstem function in babies with meningitis. Several more recent prospective studies using BAERs to evaluate auditory function in children with meningitis place the incidence of significant hearing loss in the range of 10–20 percent (Ozdamar et al., 1983; Vienny et al., 1984). Ozdamar found BAER abnormalities in 37 percent of children with bacterial meningitis tested prior to discharge from the hospital. Conductive hearing loss was the most common abnormal

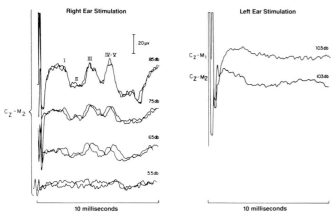

Figure 4-5. Case 2. BAERs in a 9-month-old youngster with meningitis. This 9-month-old baby presented 3 days after the onset of fever with lethargy, irritability, nuchal rigidity, and a markedly bulging fontanel. He appeared not to hear, although his marked irritability precluded adequate clinical auditory assessment. Lumbar puncture revealed cloudy cerebrospinal fluid (CSF) with 670 white cells, 99% of which were polys. The CSF protein was 100 mg.% and the CSF glucose was 2 mg.%. The baby was treated with ampicillin and chloramphenicol. Hemophilus influenza infection was subsequently identified. The course was complicated by persistent fever 2 weeks into therapy, and by bilateral subdural effusions. BAERs performed at the end of the first and third weeks showed no reponse to 103 dB stimulation on the left side and an elevated threshold on the right side. Follow-up BAER and audiometry 6 months later confirmed these results. In this case BAERs permitted the early diagnosis of significant bilateral hearing loss.

pattern, being seen in 15 percent. Twelve percent showed a pattern consistent with sensorineural hearing loss, and 8 percent showed central abnormalities. Vienny et al. serially studied 51 children with bacterial meningitis as early as 48 hours after diagnosis and weekly thereafter. While 33 percent were abnormal at first testing, only 10 percent remained abnormal at discharge. All of the 10 percent had persistent sensorineural deafness at follow-up. In neither study did a case of late deafness emerge that was not detected by early BAER testing (Case 2, Fig. 4-5).

BAERs are crucial in the auditory evaluation of babies with meningitis, patients in whom the accuracy of conventional audiometry is often questionable. BAERs permit early diagnosis of hearing impairment and permit objective assessment of the need for amplification and specific educational therapy. It is of note that BAERs as conventionally done test primarily the high-frequency spectrum of the auditory system. BAERs could fail to detect a selective low-frequency deficit, or may provide an overpessimistic appraisal of hearing in the patient with a selective high-frequency hearing loss. Vienny et al. (1984) reported 1 infant with neonatal meningitis who had no response to 90 dB stimulation but subsequently had normal language and an audiometrically demonstrated high-frequency hearing loss.

BAER IN BRAINSTEM GLIOMAS

Several series in the literature suggest that BAERs are routinely abnormal in patients with intrinsic pontine gliomas (Davis et al., 1985; Hecox et al., 1981). BAER abnormalities are clearly not specific for this entity, or for any other neurologic disease for that matter, and consist of a variety of "central" abnormalities, such as increased III–V latency, poorly formed waves IV and V, or absence of later components. These abnormalities are frequently seen prior to changes on the computed tomography (CT) scan, suggesting that BAERs are valuable in the evaluation of youngsters with clinical brainstem findings and normal CT scans (Nodar et al., 1980A; Guthkelch et al., 1985). Abnormal BAERs in a youngster with brainstem findings and normal posterior fossa CT scan would be a clear indication for MRI (magnetic resonance) scanning (Case 3, Fig. 4-6).

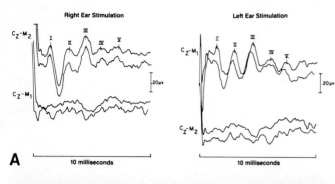

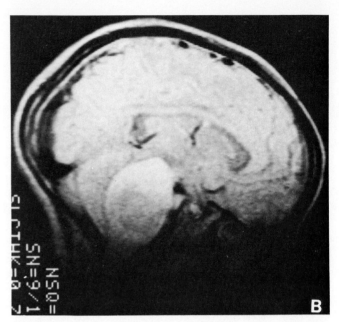

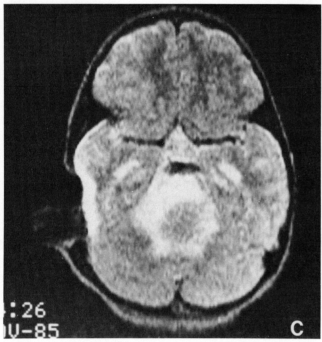

Figure 4-6. Case 3. BAERs in a 4-year-old girl evaluated for ataxia and dysarthria. This 4-year-old child was referred to the neurology clinic for a several-year history of clumsiness and dysarthric speech. On neurological exam, the child was noted to have a mild left sixth-nerve palsy, significant dysarthria, truncal and appendicular ataxia, and bilateral Babinski's signs. The CT scan showed an enhancing posterior fossa mass. The enclosed MRI scan reveals an enhancing intrinsic pontine lesion which proved to be brainstem glioma. BAERs in this youngster showed bilaterally prolonged I–V interpeak latencies with abnormal morphology and amplitude of waves IV and V consistent with diffuse brainstem disease.

BAER IN NEURODEGENERATIVE DISEASE

BAERs are often significantly abnormal in the primary white matter diseases of the brain such as Pelizaeus-Merzbacher, metachromatic leukodystrophy, and Leigh's disease and, along with the electroencephalogram (EEG), help differentiate grey from white matter disease in the young child. Patients with Pelizaeus-Merzbacher disease have abnormal BAERS, often with no potentials recordable after waves I and II, even in the first month of life when their neurological exams may be normal apart from mild nystagmus (Garg et al., 1983). Abnormal BAERs have also been recorded in patients with metachromatic leukodystrophy and adrenoleukodystrophy with a variety of central transmission abnormalities seen, depending on the severity of clinical illness. Abnormal BAERS have been reported with marked frequency in Leigh's disease. Abnormalities of wave V, and increased I–V latencies, are most often described and are seen even before CT scan abnormalities are noted (Davis et al., 1985) (Cases 4 and 5, Figs. 4-7 and 4-8).

BAER IN COMA AND BRAIN DEATH

The extent of neuronal damage may be difficult to assess in the comatose patient on clinical grounds. The electroencephalogram may be influenced by treatment modalities for brain resuscitation, and a CT scan is inadequate in the assessment of the physiologic integrity of the brainstem. BAERs have been suggested as having a unique role in the evaluation of the comatose patient (Garg et al., 1983). Goitein et al. (1983) noted in a group of comatose youngsters, that regardless of the etiology or depth of coma, recovery occurred in all patients with normal BAERs and death occurred in all patients with the absence of all BAER components. Intermediate central abnormalities (increased I–V latency, amplitude ratio abnormalities, etc.) were associated with variable outcomes. Changes in serial BAERs reliably predicted or paralleled clinical change, in the hands of these researchers, but others seriously question the prognostic ability of the BAER (see Chapter 3).

As an objective measure of brainstem integrity, BAERs have also been proposed as an important adjunctive diagnostic

Right Ear Stimulation

Left Ear Stimulation

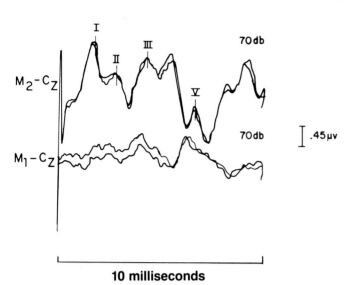

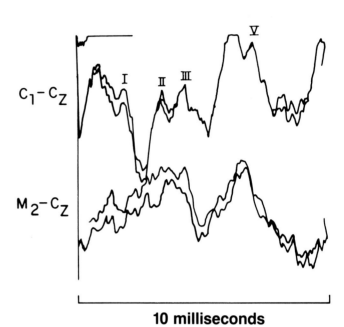

10 milliseconds

Figure 4-7. Case 4. This $2\frac{1}{2}$ year old youngster presented with a history of regression in neurological function following a viral illness at 15 months. The physical exam revealed nystagmus, chorea, and ataxia. The patient was acidotic, and MRI scan revealed changes in the brainstem consistent with Leigh's disease. Brainstem auditory evoked responses show increased I–V interpeak latency (greater than 5.0 msec) bilaterally and an abnormal wave V : wave I amplitude ratio to right ear stimulation. (Courtesy of Dr. Darryl C. DeVivo).

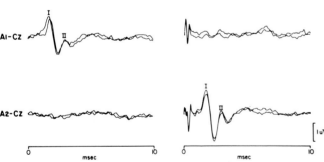

Figure 4-8. Case 5. This 14-month-old male was evaluated for irregular nystagmus, head-rolling, and mildly delayed motor development. The patient had a brother, age 7, who exhibited nystagmus, spastic diplegia, and optic atrophy. The clinical diagnosis was that of Pelizaeus-Merzbacher disease. BAEPs characteristically demonstrate disappearance of later waves (III, IV, and V) seen in the leukodystrophies and other demyelinating states.

tool in the determination of pediatric brain death (Goitein et al., 1983). Steinhart and Weiss (1985) studied 10 children who met the clinical and electroencephalographic criteria of brain death, and 13 comatose youngsters who did not meet those criteria. Nine of the 10 clinically brain dead children had absent BAERs and in one, only wave I was recorded. In comatose youngsters who did not meet the brain death criteria, at least 2 waves were present. Goldie et al. (1981), in their study of brain death in both children and adults, noted the absence of all BAER components in 77 percent of patients meeting the clinical and electroencephalographic criteria of brain death. They postulated that the cessation of intracranial circulation caused destruction of the eighth nerve and loss of wave I. However, in the absence of wave I, it is impossible to be certain that the peripheral auditory apparatus is adequately functional to allow brainstem stimulation. In addition, Taylor et al. (1983) reported a 33-month-old infant with a severe hypoxic ischemic encephalopathy who did not meet the full clinical and electroencephalographic criteria of brain death, but who lost all BAER components. This youngster subsequently recovered most of the BAER waves and survived, although in the vegetative state. The authors suggest that the loss of BAERs may be reversible and cannot be used in isolation as a criterion for brain death. In this case, the absence of wave I raises the question of a peripheral auditory factor in the etiology of the loss of BAER components especially in near-drowning victims (Owen & Lai, 1984). In conclusion, the frequent finding (90 percent of Steinhart's clinically brain dead patients) of the loss of all BAER components and the consequent uncertainty about the role of peripheral factors significantly limit the utility of BAERs in the determination of brain death. On the positive side, BAERs are notoriously resistant to anesthetic levels of various agents used in "brain resuscitation." They can provide means of following comatose patients when the clinical and electroencephalographic evaluation is precluded by high-dose barbiturate therapy (Case 6, Fig. 4-9).

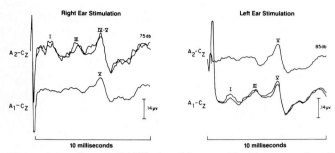

Figure 4-9. Case 6. BAERs in a 13-year-old with severe closed head injury. This 13-year-old youngster presented after a severe closed head injury with decerebrate posturing to painful stimuli and intact brainstem reflexes. A CT scan showed cerebral edema. The patient was treated with anesthetic doses of pentobarbital. Within the next 24 hours, he lost oculocephalic, pupillary, and corneal reflexes and was considered to be "brain dead." BAERs in this youngster showed a slightly prolonged I–V interpeak latency, but the presence of central conduction showed that clearly this youngster would not meet the BAER criteria for brain death. The patient has made an incomplete recovery. BAERs in this case were minimally abnormal and demonstrated the persistence of central auditory conduction. The BAER preservation suggested that the barbiturates were responsible for the loss of brainstem reflexes on clinical exam.

whom conventional audiometry often yields inconclusive results at best. Several recent studies have shown a slight increase in central transmission time in autistic youngsters, suggesting a central auditory deficit as the etiology of the language impairment in these youngsters (Sohmer and Student, 1978; Skoff et al., 1980; Taylor et al., 1982). Just as important, these studies have also demonstrated a significant incidence of unrecognized hearing loss in autistic youngsters.

Within a series of children less than 2 years of age referred for BAERs as part of a neurologic evaluation, 20 percent had unrecognized hearing disorders severe enough to require additional evaluation for amplification (Hecox et al., 1981). Clearly, threshold testing is mandatory in all nonverbal youngsters referred for BAERs (Case 7, Fig. 4-10).

CONCLUSION

BAERs can be reliably recorded with relative ease even in a small pre-term infant. There are no BAER abnormalities pathognomonic of a particular neurologic disease entity. Their major use in pediatric neurologic practice lies in:

1. the identification, characterization, and quantification of hearing loss in children unable to cooperate for conventional audiometry by virtue of age or neurologic impairment
2. the objective assessment of brainstem function in youngsters with diffuse cerebral dysfunction suspected of having a white matter disease where brainstem dysfunction is prominent (as in Leigh's disease, or Pelizaeus-Merzbacher disease)

BAER IN THE ASSESSMENT OF PEDIATRIC HEARING LOSS

BAER recording is the most reliable method of estimating auditory sensitivity in infants, young children, and uncooperative patients. The weakest auditory stimulus that produces a consistent wave V response establishes the threshold but does not ensure the presence of the cortical event of "hearing." The determination of a latency-intensity graph in a youngster with an elevated auditory threshold helps to identify the nature of the auditory impairment. In a youngster with conductive hearing loss, the patient's latency-intensity curve parallels, but is displaced from, the normal curve. The degree of displacement from the normal curve is a measure of the amount of hearing loss. In youngsters with sensorineural hearing loss, the latency-intensity curve differs in that the more the signal intensity exceeds the threshold, the less the difference between the normal and abnormal curves. The latency-intensity curve eventually intersects and joins the normal curve.

Of note is the fact that a child whose hearing impairment is restricted to the low frequencies may have an entirely normal BAER. The BAER method of hearing assessment can fail to detect a loss limited to frequencies below 1000Hz. Stimulation with tone bursts may permit the evaluation of lower-frequency hearing losses (Davis and Owen, 1985) (Chapter 2).

BAERs are of particular usefulness in testing hyperactive, autistic, and multiply handicapped youngsters, patients in

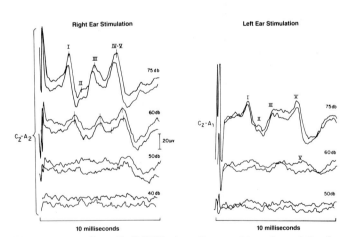

Figure 4-10. Case 7. BAERs in a 2-year-old evaluated for delayed language. This 2-year-old youngster was evaluated for clumsiness and delayed expressive and receptive language function. On exam, he was a hyperactive child with a clumsy gait and virtually no expressive language function. BAERs demonstrated an elevated threshold bilaterally, consistent with conductive hearing loss. Followup BAERs after treatment for serous otitis were normal. The youngster is presently enrolled in a program for the language impaired and has made slight progress. The BAERs in this instance identified a conductive deficit.

3. the confirmation and localization of brainstem dysfunction in patients with clinical brainstem findings, i.e., brainstem glioma suspects. This provides a physiologic adjunct to radiologic studies (CT and MRI).

REFERENCES

Bradford, BC, Baudin, J, Conway, MJ, et al. (1985). Identification of sensory neural hearing loss in very pre-term infants by brain stem auditory evoked potentials. *Arch Dis Child, 60*, 105–109

Davis, H, Owen, J (1985). *Auditory evoked potential testing, clinical applications* (p. 55). Florida: Grune & Stratton

Davis, SL, Aminoff, MJ, Berg, BO (1985). Brain stem auditory evoked potentials in children with brain stem or cerebellar dysfunction. *Arch Neurol, 42*, 156–160

Despland, PA, Galambos, R (1980). The auditory brain stem response is a useful diagnostic tool in the intensive care nursery. *Pediat Res, 14*, 154–163

Despland, PA, Galambos, R (1982). The brain stem auditory evoked potential is a useful diagnostic tool in evaluating risk factors for hearing loss in neonatology. In J Corjon, F Mauguiere, & M Revol (Eds.) *Clinical applications of evoked potentials in neurology* (p. 241). New York: Raven Press

Garg, BP, Markand, ON, DeMyer, WE (1983). Usefulness of BAER studies in the early diagnosis of Pelizaeus-Merzbacher disease. *Neurology, 33*, 955–958

Goitein, KJ, Amit, Y, Fainmesser, P, Sohmer, H (1983). Diagnostic and prognostic value of auditory nerve brain stem evoked potentials, evoked responses in comatose children. *Crit Care Med, 11*, 91–94

Goldie, WD, Khiappa, KH, Young, RR, et al. (1981). Brain stem auditory and short latency somatosensory evoked responses in brain death. *Neurology, 31*, 248–256

Gupta, PR, Guilleminault, C, Dorfman, LJ (1981). Brain stem auditory evoked potentials in near-miss sudden infant death syndrome. *J Pediatr, 98*, 791–794

Guthkelch, AN, Vries, JK, Sclabassi, RJ (1985). Early detection of brainstem giona using brainstem auditory evoked potential. *Developmental medicine and child neurology, 27* (p. 331)

Hecox, KE, Come, B (1981). Prognostic importance of brain stem auditory evoked responses after asphyxia. *Neurology, 31*, 1429–1434

Hecox, KE, Come, B, Blaw, ME (1981). Brain stem auditory evoked response in the diagnosis of pediatric neurologic disease. *Neurology, 31*, 832–840

Hecox, K, Burkard, R (1982). Developmental dependencies of the human brain stem auditory evoked response. *Ann NY Acad Sci, 388*, 538–556

Luders, H, Orlowski, J, Dinner, D, et al. (1984). Fairfield auditory evoked potentials in near miss sudden infant death syndrome. *Arch Neurol, 41*, 615–17

Lutschg, J, Pfenninger, J, et al. (1983). Brain stem auditory evoked potentials and early somatosensory evoked potentials in neural intensively treated comatose children. *Am J Dis Child, 137*, 421–426

Mochizuki, Y, Go, T, Ohkubo, H, et al. (1982). Developmental changes of brain stem auditory evoked potentials in normal human subjects from infants to young adults. *Brain Dev, 4*, 127–136

Nodar, RH, Hahn, J, Levine, HL (1980). Brain stem auditory evoked potentials in determining the site of a lesion of brain stem gliomas in children. *Laryngoscope, 90*, 258–266

Nodar, RH, Lonsdale, D, Orlowski, JP (1980B). Abnormal brain stem potentials in infants with threatened sudden infant death syndrome. *Head Neck Surg, 88*, 619–621

Ochs, R, Markand, ON, DeMyer, WE (1979). Brain stem auditory evoked responses in leukodystrophies. *Neurology, 29*, 1089–1093

Orlowski, JP, Nodar, RH, Lonsdale, D (1979). Abnormal brain stem auditory evoked potentials in infants with threatened sudden infant death syndrome. *Cleve C Q, 46*, 77–82

Owen, J, Lai, CW (1984). Letter to the editor. *N Engl J Med, 310*, 246

Ozdamar, O, Kraus, N, Stein, L (1983). Auditory brain stem responses in infants recovering from meningitis. *Arch Otolaryngol, 109*, 13–18

Roberts, JL, Davis, H, Phon, GL, et al. (1982). Auditory brain stem responses in preterm neonates, maturation and followup. *J Pediatr, 101*, 257–263

Salamy, A, McKean, CM (1976). Postnatal development of human brain stem potential during the first year of life. *Electroencephalogr Clin Neurophysiol, 40*, 418–426

Skoff, BF, Mirsky, AF, Turner, D (1980). Prolonged brain stem transmission time in autism. *Psychiatry Res, 2*, 157–167

Sohmer, H, Student, M (1978). Auditory nerve and brain stem evoked responses in normal autistic minimal brain dysfunction and cycle motor retarded children. *Electroencephalogr Clin Neurophysiol, 44*, 380–388

Starr, A, Amlie, RN, Martin, WH, Sanders, S (1977). Development of auditory function in newborn infants revealed by auditory brain stem potentials. *Pediatrics, 60*, 831–839

Stein, L, Ozdamar, O, et al. (1983). Followup of infants screened by auditory brain stem response in the neonatal intensive care unit. *J Pediatr, 103*, 447–453

Steinhart, CM, Weiss, IP (1985). Use of brain stem auditory evoked potentials in pediatric brain death. *Crit Care Med, 13*, 560–562

Stockard, JW, Westmoreland, BF (1981). Technical considerations in the recording and interpretation of brain stem auditory evoked potential for neonatal neurologic diagnosis. *Am J EEG Technol, 21*, 31–54

Stockard, JJ (1982). Brain stem auditory evoked potentials in adult and infant sleep apnea syndromes including sudden infant death syndrome and near miss for sudden infant death. *Ann NY Acad Sci, 388*, 433–463

Stockard, JW, Stockard, JJ, et al. (1983). Prognostic value of brain stem auditory evoked potentials in neonates. *Arch Neurol, 40*, 360–365

Swartz, MN, Dodge, PR (1965). Bacterial meningitis. A review of selected aspects—General clinical features, special problems complications and clinical pathologic correlations. *N Engl J Med, 272*, 954–962

Taylor, MJ, Rosenblatt, B, Linschoten, L (1982). Auditory brain stem response abnormalities in autistic children. *Can J Neurol Sci, 9*, 429–433

Taylor, MJ, Houston, BD, Lowry, NJ (1983). Recovery of auditory brain stem responses after a severe hypoxic ischemic insult. *N Engl J Med, 309*, 1169–70

Vienny, H, Despland, PA, Lutschg, J, et al. (1984). Early diagnosis and evolution of deafness in childhood bacterial meningitis. A study using brain stem auditory evoked potentials. *Pediatrics, 73*, 579–586

James W. Hall III
Denise A. Tucker

5

The Auditory Brainstem Response in Acute Brain Injury

Rational management of the acute, brain-injured patient requires systematic monitoring of neurologic status. Structural central nervous system (CNS) damage can be documented with computerized tomography (CT). CT, however, cannot be done at the bedside, and is, therefore, not a feasible technique for CNS monitoring. In addition, CT does not provide information on the functional status of neurons. Continuous measurement of systemic physiologic parameters, and CNS physiologic parameters, such as mean arterial pressure (MAP), intracranial pressure (ICP), and blood gases (PaO_2, $PaCO_2$) by means of monitoring devices provides valuable data for determining the status of the neuronal environment, and for preventing CNS ischemia and hypoxia (Messick et al., 1985; Miller, et al., 1977; Nordby and Gunnerod, 1985; Saul and Decker, 1982). Still, although clinically indispensible, these parameters do not reflect integrity of neurons in specific regions of the CNS but, rather, overall status. Finally, the clinical neurological examination is the mainstay of CNS monitoring in this patient population. Unfortunately, the neurological examination has several crucial limitations. Neurologic signs may be invalidated by therapy modalities commonly employed in acutely brain-injured patients, such as chemical paralyzers and high-dose barbiturates (Marshall et al., 1979; Messick et al., 1985; Nordby and Nesbakken, 1984; Piatt and Schiff, 1984; Rockoff, 1984; Ward et al., 1985). Furthermore, localization of lesions in the comatose patient is often not possible solely on the basis of the neurological examination.

There is, therefore, the need for a method of objectively and regularly assessing CNS functional status, a method that meets at least 9 clinically important criteria:

1. Mobility. Assessment can be carried out at bedside in an intensive care unit (ICU) environment. Transportation of acute brain-injured patients increases the risk of CNS damage and is a clear contraindication for a monitoring technique.
2. Noninvasiveness. Repeated measurement does not require insertion of needles or catheters.
3. Safety. The technique does not pose substantial risk or harm to the patient, and does not involve radioactive substances.
4. Limited time. Assessment can be completed in a reasonable period of time, e.g., 1 hour or less, so as not to interfere with ongoing intensive care of the patient.
5. Objectivity. The test data can be stored for later analyses, and be subjected to mathematical and/or statistical manipulation.
6. Sensitivity. The technique is sensitive to subtle changes in neuronal functional status.
7. Specificity. The information obtained may not be limited to a specific anatomical region, yet does provide information on specific regions of the CNS.
8. Coma/therapy independence. The test results are not seriously influenced by the level of coma, nor by commonly used medical therapy modalities, such as sedatives, paralyzers, hyperosmolar drugs, and barbiturates.
9. Cost. Testing fees must be reasonable.

The auditory evoked responses (AERs), in particular the auditory brainstem evoked response (ABR), and sensory evoked

Clinical Atlas of Auditory Evoked Potentials
ISBN 0-8089-1896-6

responses (SERs) in general, meet these clinically important criteria, and have multiple applications in acutely brain-injured patients. Perhaps the first clinical reports of the application of multimodality SERs in acutely brain-injured patients were the papers published by Greenberg and his colleagues in the 1970s (Greenberg and Becker, 1976; Greenberg et al., 1977). These important clinical studies generated considerable interest in the potential value of SERs in this population, and provided the impetus for our initial attempts to measure evoked responses in the ICU.

In this chapter, we will demonstrate with original clinical data the use of SERs in monitoring CNS status in the ICU, and the factors that must be considered for meaningful interpretation of SER findings. The clinical data and experiences that we present are based on a combined caseload of over 900 acutely injured adult and pediatric patients with a variety of brain pathologies. All data were collected at bedside in an ICU environment with commercially available equipment (Nicolet CA-1000 evoked response system). Although the emphasis is on the ABR, we will also describe the relationship among the evoked response stimulus modalities in the acutely brain-injured population. We will present illustrations of clinical applications with actual case reports and support these observations with group data when available. Finally, we will stress the incorporation of SER information into the more traditional CNS monitoring database, describing the relationship of evoked reponse outcome to neurological signs, physiologic parameters, neuroradiographic information, and the relationship among the evoked response stimulus modalities.

FACTORS INFLUENCING EVOKED RESPONSES IN THE ICU

ARTIFACT IN ABR MEASUREMENT

Environmental electrical artifact is probably the most troublesome and commonly encountered obstacle to obtaining reliable and meaningful evoked response data in an ICU environment. There are many sources of electrical artifact, including 60Hz line noise and a spectrum of airborne electromagnetic energies. However, although an ICU is a potentially hostile environment for evoked response recording, it is possible to routinely measure evoked responses for auditory, somatosensory, and visual stimulus modalities from acutely, severely brain-injured children and adults with commercially available equipment.

Precautions for minimizing the deleterious effects of electrical artifact include reliance on well-grounded evoked response measurement instrumentation, quality electrodes, low interelectrode resistance (less than 5000 ohm), and, especially, a very good electrical contact for the ground electrode. Guidelines for optimizing evoked response recording in the ICU have been recently published (Hall et al., 1985A; Hall and Tucker, 1985; Hall and Tucker, 1986). As a last resort, we attempt to reduce artifact contamination by restricting the neural filter setting, e.g., from 30–3000Hz to 150–1500Hz for the ABR and, if that technique fails, returning to the patient's bedside at another time, perhaps in the evening.

Neuromuscular artifact is a less serious problem in the acute period following brain injury than during recovery. As we note below, the patient is typically sedated, often paralyzed chemically, and sometimes in deep, barbiturate-induced coma. During recovery from injury, however, increasing movement can contribute to muscular artifact that contaminates or even precludes evoked response recording. Muscle artifact is a more significant factor for the auditory middle-latency response and somatosensory responses (SERs) than for the ABR. Sometimes it is necessary to request mild sedation in patients recovering from brain injury in order to successfully carry out testing.

OTOLOGIC PATHOLOGY

Peripheral auditory abnormalities associated with otologic pathology must be regularly considered in the interpretation of auditory evoked responses recorded from traumatically head-injured patients and from brain-injured patients with other etiologies, such as meningitis. The frequent occurrence of auditory abnormalities following head trauma is well-recognized (Aguilar et al., 1986; Hall et al., 1982; Hall et al., 1983a,b). Two-thirds of the patients in our ICU were found to have otologic pathology by physical examination (Aguilar et al., 1986). Hemotympanum was most common (33 percent). Prolonged coma and mechanical ventilation may contribute to the development of middle-ear pathology associated with eustachian tube dysfunction and middle-ear pressure abnormalities (Hall et al., 1982) and lead to conductive hearing loss, usually transient. Documentation of middle-ear status must be done on an ongoing basis whenever AER changes suggest peripheral otologic pathology during the acute period in the ICU. Failure to take peripheral auditory deficits into account in the interpretation of the ABR may confound interpretation of serial findings and result in incorrect inferences about CNS status. Taylor, Houston, and Lowry (1983) presented a case report of a brain-injured child monitored with the ABR. The ABR at one point disappeared and then reappeared. The child survived. The authors offered the case as evidence that the ABR is not a reliable measure of CNS status in this population, and interpretation of the loss of an ABR as a sign of severe neurologic dysfunction is not advisable clinically. After close scrutiny of their findings, however, we would conclude that the disappearance of the ABR was not due to dynamic brainstem pathology but, rather, to transient peripheral otologic pathology. Even the wave I was not observed at one point, and this finding occurred after increased wave I latencies were noted. We have stressed the importance of documenting middle-ear function with otologic examination, immittance audiometry, and bone-conduction ABR stimulation as a routine practice in acute brain injury (Hall et al., 1982; Hall and Mackey-Hargadine, 1984; Aguilar et al., 1986).

As a rule, AER assessment in the ICU is done for evaluation of CNS status. Therefore, we usually present auditory stimulation only at high intensity levels (75–95 dB HL re: click threshold). Techniques for enhancing AER waveforms in patients with apparent otologic pathology include the use of insert acoustic transducers when bandages cover the ears, bone-conduction stimulation when severe middle-ear dysfunction is suspected, and multi-channel recordings (Aguilar et al., 1986; Hall et al., 1984B; Hall and Mackey-Hargadine, 1984; Hall et al., 1985A; Hall and Tucker, 1985).

Among these modifications of standard measurement techniques, multi-channel recordings are especially useful. The application of a four-channel, multi-channel electrode array in detection of ABR wave components is illustrated by the following case report.

Case 1

The patient was a 23-year-old male involved in an accident while driving a truck. He was thrown from the vehicle, sustaining a head injury. Following helicopter transport from an outlying hospital to the Hermann Hospital emergency room (HHER), the patient remained unconscious. He was taken to CT scanning, which showed severe cerebral swelling, with a large left-to-right shift (Fig. 5-1). Upon arrival at the ICU, neurologic status was poor. Pupils were bilaterally pinpoint. There were very sluggish corneal and doll's eyes (oculocephalic) responses, and extensor posturing to deep pain. Glasgow coma scale (GCS) was 4. Monitored ICP was 70 mmHg. Maximum medical therapy was initiated, including hyperventilation, mannitol, and a bolus of pentobarbital. Blood pressure (systolic) decreased to below 80 mmHg.

Initial AER assessment was carried out within 12 hours of hospital admission with neurologic status as described above. There was a reliable, well-formed ABR for right-ear stimulation as, illustrated in Figure 5-2. Left-ear stimulation at maximum stimulation level (95 dB) failed to generate a clear response with the usual electrode array (forehead-to-stimulus ipsilateral earlobe electrode pair). Blood was noted in the left ear canal and on the pinna. We then recorded the ABR with a four-channel electrode array (see Hall et al., 1984B for technical details). As seen in Figure 5-2, the forehead-noncephalic electrode combination appeared to resolve a small-amplitude but repeatable wave V component, and the contralateral-to-ipsilateral earlobe (i.e., horizontal) array produced small wave I and III components. Calculating interwave latencies from these components resulted in an interpretation of caudal brainstem transmission time delay on the left, and normal brainstem transmission time on the right. The patient's neurological condition and ABR progressively deteriorated over the course of the next 10 days, with brain death occurring on the 11th post-injury day. The traditional single-channel electrode array is, in our experience, adequate for the vast majority of ABR recordings in the acutely brain-injured population. Occasionally, however, application of a multichannel electrode array seems to enhance detection of wave components and aids in the meaningful interpretation of ABR findings.

BODY TEMPERATURE

Evaluating a patient with a low body temperature is a condition frequently encountered in the operating room (OR) and ICU. Mild hypothermia often occurs in a variety of surgical procedures. Moderate to deep hypothermia is induced in cardiovascular surgery. In the ICU, hypothermia can be seen in patients who have suffered cardiac arrest. Additionally, patients with brainstem pathology often demonstrate an inability to regulate their body temperature. Acute care therapies, such as barbiturate coma, may also lower temperature.

Hypothermia has a profound effect on evoked response testing. Rosenblum, Ruth, and Gal (1985) reported that intervals between ABR waves I–V increased during topical cooling in cardiopulmonary bypass surgery. In their study, the I–V interval reached 9.2 msec at 15°C, and wave I could still be recorded at 14°C. Wave V was difficult to identify below 15°C. Marshall and Donchin (1981) found that the reduction of 1°C in body temperature corresponded to a 0.2 msec increase in the latency of wave V.

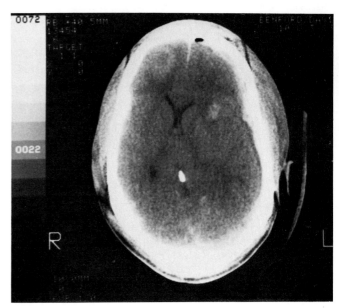

Figure 5-1. Computerized tomography for a 23-year-old male with severe closed head injury (Case 1). Right side of brain is on left side of CT for this figure and subsequent figures, unless otherwise noted.

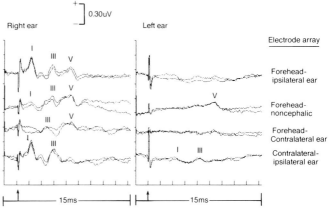

Figure 5-2. Auditory brainstem response (ABR) waveforms recorded simultaneously with four-channel electrode array for Case 1. Note enhancement of wave components on left with multiple channels.

Visually evoked responses (VERs) are also sensitive to body temperature. Russ et al. (1984) found that the major negative and positive VER components lengthened with decreasing temperatures. They also reported that VER waveforms disappeared at different temperature levels, depending on the rapidity of cooling. They found that VER components recovered immediately during rewarming. Reilly et al. (1978) studied the effects of hypothermia on VERs in children. They reported that the latency of the P2 peak became much more variable than the N1 component at low body temperatures, suggesting that the N1 component may be more useful in following the effects of CNS stresses in pediatric patients.

Kopf et al. (1985) found that somatosensory conduction time between N13 and N20 increased from 6.4 msec to 10.3 msec during hypothermia, with an increase in conduction time of 6.6 percent for a 1°C drop in the esophageal temperature. Coles et al. (1984) studied serial SERs (SSERs) in 9 infants during clinical procedures involving profound hypothermic circulatory arrest. They found that cortical evoked potentials disappeared below 18°C and remained absent throughout the period of circulatory arrest. Their study demonstrated that neurologic complications were not reflected in intraoperative SER.

Case 2

The patient was a 12-year-old male admitted to the Northwest Texas Hospital (NWTH) pediatric ICU after having a seizure and losing consciousness. At admission, he was comatose and responsive to noxious stimuli only. Pupils were 6–7 mm and reactive to light. Body temperature was 103°F. A CT scan revealed diffuse cerebral edema. The patient was hyperventilated and given mannitol and albumin. He was also started on phenobarbital to reduce cerebral metabolism, in an attempt to protect the brain from possible ischemia. Drug screens, blood culture, and a lumbar puncture were all normal. Diagnosis was viral encephalitis.

The first set of multi-modality evoked responses tests was carried out on the day of admission. Body temperature at that time was 100°F. Repeat studies were carried out twice on the second day. The first set was obtained when temperature had decreased to 92°F. The patient was placed on a heating blanket to raise his temperature, and evoked response measures were again made when temperature had returned to 100°F. A fourth and final set of data was obtained the next day when temperature had remained stable for 24 hours.

The neural conduction time between waves I and V in the ABR was delayed when the patient was hypothermic, but all the waveforms remained present (Fig. 5-3). The I–V latencies returned to normal after the body temperature stabilized. The visual evoked response showed a mild delay initially upon admission and a moderate delay when the patient was hypothermic. Even when the patient's temperature returned to normal, however, the VER continued to worsen, until finally there were no apparent waveform components. With decreased and then increased temperature, the median nerve SSER latencies increased substantially and then returned to normal, similar to the ABR data. Amplitude of the SSER did not return to normal, however, when the temperature had stabilized (Fig. 5-4).

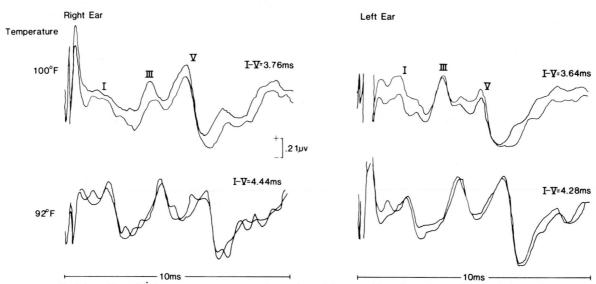

Figure 5-3. Serial auditory brainstem response waveforms for a 12-year-old male with viral encephalitis (Case 2). Note increased interwave latencies at lower temperatures (see Table 5-1).

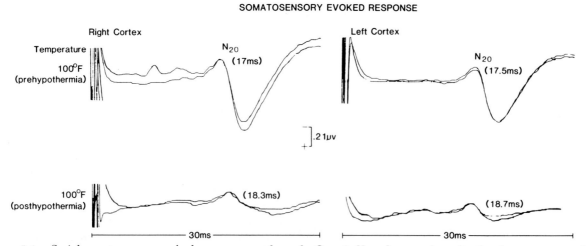

Figure 5-4. Serial somatosensory evoked response waveforms for Case 2. Note decreased amplitude after temperature had returned to normal.

The patient survived and regained consciousness after several weeks of hospital stay. His speaking and walking ability are intact, but he has demonstrated major difficulties in returning to a normal school routine. He reports problems in memory and in working math problems. This case illustrates the importance of taking temperature into account in interpreting SERs, particularly serial recordings. It is sometimes difficult to differentiate SER changes that are temperature related from those that reflect pathophysiologic processes. The combined use of multimodalities may help in this differentiation.

THERAPEUTIC MODALITIES

Therapeutic modalities commonly used in the management of acute brain injury, as noted above, may compromise the validity of the clinical neurologic examination. For the most part, these same drugs do not seriously affect the ABR. Among the therapeutic modalities that do not appear to influence the ABR are chemical paralyzing agents (e.g., Pavulon, Metacurine), sedatives (e.g., Haldol, morphine), therapeutic doses of anti-convulsants (e.g., Dilantin) and barbiturates (e.g., high-dose pentobarbital) (Hall et al., 1985A; Hall, 1985; Marsh, et al., 1984; Newlon et al., 1983; Samra et al., 1985; Sutton et al., 1982). The possible effect of other therapies, such as hyperosmolar drugs, has not, to our knowledge, been investigated. The differential influence of high-dose barbiturates on the ABR versus auditory middle-latency response (AMR) is illustrated by the following case report.

Case 3: Barbiturate Coma

A 26-year-old male was involved in a motor vehicle accident (MVA) and found unconscious outside his automobile. Glasgow Coma Scale score was 3. He was taken to an outlying hospital where he was given emergency therapy (intubation and hyperventilation). Upon the arrival of the Life Flight helicopter, the patient was unresponsive to painful stimuli. Both pupils were reactive. He was bleeding from the left ear. On arrival at the HHER emergency room, neurologic status had improved. He was opening his eyes on command and moving purposefully. GCS was 13. The improvement followed treatment with mannitol and Decadron and was also attributed to reduced effect of alcohol and recreational drugs.

On the first day post-injury, the patient's neurologic status deteriorated abruptly. Pupils were dilated bilaterally, and he was decerebrate. Emergency CT scan showed diffuse subarachnoid hemorrhage and infarction in the distribution of the anterior cerebral arteries. At placement of an ICP monitor, opening pressure was 35 cm H_2O. During the course of the next 2 weeks, there were recurrent elevations of ICP that did not respond to traditional medical therapy, and barbiturate coma was induced. Upon return to the ICU following placement of the ICP monitor, the ABR and AMR were normal bilaterally (Fig. 5-5). Throughout the barbiturate coma, we recorded a well-formed, reliable ABR. The AMR, in contrast, was suppressed by high blood levels of barbiturates.

This case typifies our experience with AERs in barbiturate coma. The ABR appears to be remarkably resistant to the CNS suppressant effect of barbiturates, whereas the AMR is very sensitive to even relatively low doses of the drug, resulting in blood levels of 10 μg/ml or less. The independence of the ABR with respect to barbiturates is a major clinical advantage, as we will demonstrate in this chapter.

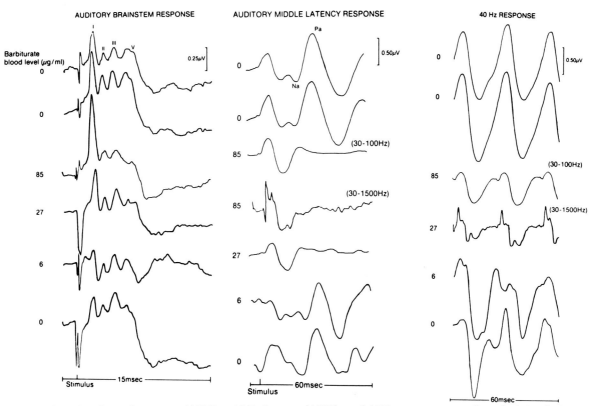

Figure 5-5. Serial auditory brainstem (ABR), middle-latency (AMR), and 40Hz response recordings before, during, and after barbiturate coma for a 26-year-old male with closed head injury (Case 3).

RELATIONSHIPS AMONG ABR AND OTHER NEURODIAGNOSTIC FINDINGS

CLINICAL NEUROLOGIC FINDINGS

Previous reports of the ABR and neurologic findings describe good clinical correlations. Uziel and Benezech (1978) found clear-cut relationships among ABR abnormalities and brainstem signs. Patients with dilated and unreactive pupils, for example, were considered to have pontine or lower-brainstem lesions, and typically showed marked ABR alterations, including wave III and V abnormalities. Tsubokawa and colleagues (1980) reported similar correlations. Although ABR abnormalities were occasionally noted in patients without clinical brainstem deficits, they postulated that this setting might predict impending progressive brainstem dysfunction. Gross ABR abnormalities, such as disappearance of waves III and/or V, were usually found in patients with mesencephalic/pontine or lower CNS clinical signs. Our experience does not entirely support these relations between the ABR and clinical signs.

The GCS is a widely accepted method for grading depth of coma and severity of brain injury (Jennett and Teasdale, 1981). As indicated in Figure 5-6, the GCS consists of 3 measures of patient response, an eye opening, a motor, and a verbal response. The scale ranges from a low score of 3 to a high score of 15. Severe brain injury and coma is defined as a score of 8 or less. For the purpose of assessing its relationship with other neurodiagnostic findings, the ABR was graded as either normal, abnormal (wave I–V delay or absent wave V), or as no response (wave I component only or no observable components). The waveforms characterizing these grades are illustrated in Figure 5-7. The ABR/GCS relationship was assessed for 133 brain-injured patients and is summarized in Table 5-1. Although the greatest proportion of patients with an abnormal or no ABR had GCSs of 3 or 4, there was even a larger proportion of patients with a normal ABR at this GCS level. Statistically, there is no correlation between ABR and GCS. A well-formed ABR with brainstem transmission times within normal limits can be repeatedly recorded from patients with no response to deep painful stimuli. This point will be demonstrated in several of the following case reports and is a common finding in the severely brain-injured population.

Glasgow Coma Scale

Eye Opening			Total Glasgow Coma Scale Points
	Spontaneous	4	
	To Voice	3	
	To Pain	2	14-15=**5**
	None	1	11-13=**4**
Verbal Response	Oriented	5	8-10=**3**
	Confused	4	5- 7=**2**
	Inappropriate Words	3	3- 4=**1**
	Incomprehensible Words	2	
	None	1	
Motor Response	Obeys Command	6	
	Localizes Pain	5	
	Withdraw (pain)	4	
	Flexion (pain)	3	
	Extension (pain)	2	
	None	1	
Total Trauma Score			**1-16**

Figure 5-6. Glasgow Coma Scale (GCS) used in grading severity of injury and depth of coma. (See Jennett and Teasdale, 1981, for details.)

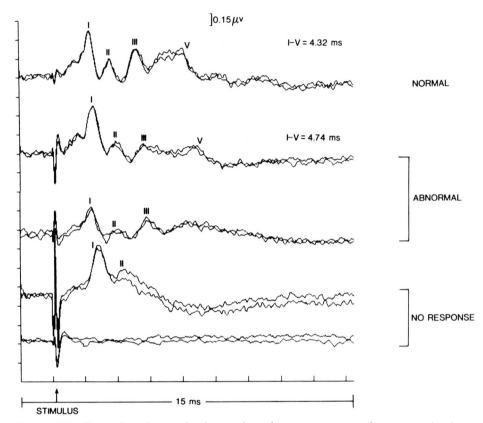

Figure 5-7. Examples of normal, abnormal, and no-response waveform categories in severely brain-injured patients. These categories are used in discussion of group data to follow.

Table 5-1 Relationship Between Initial
Glasgow Coma Scale (GCS) Score and
Initial Auditory Brainstem Response
(ABR) Findings for 114 Acute
Head-Injured Patients.

ABR	GCS		
	3 to 4	5 to 7	8 to 15
Normal	26	36	13
Abnormal*	13	7	2
No response	10	6	1

* Wave I to V latency interval greater than 2.5 standard deviations above mean value for clinical normative data

For many brain-injured patients in the ICU, particularly those managed with sedatives, chemical paralyzers, or even low doses of barbiturates, the neurologic examination is limited to evaluation of the pupillary response to light stimuli. This neurologic parameter is the most commonly reported sign in patient flow charts at our institutions. In Figure 5-8, we compare the proportion of normal versus abnormal (and no response) ABR findings in patients with pupils that are reactive and those with unreactive pupils (total N of 111). Pupillary findings were noted at the time of ABR testing. Not unexpectedly, a high proportion of patients with normal pupillary findings also had a normal ABR (79 percent) but among the patients with abnormal pupils, a majority also yielded normal ABRs. There was no statistically significant correlation between these two neurodiagnostic parameters. As we will describe with case reports to follow, abnormal pupillary responses are not invariably associated with impending neurologic decompensation. The ABR may offer evidence of brainstem integrity and the rationale for aggressive intensive management.

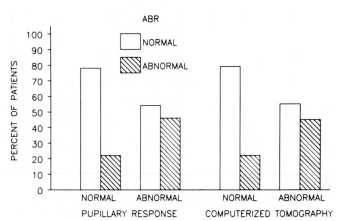

Figure 5-8. Comparison of auditory brainstem response (ABR), pupillary response, and computerized tomography (CT) findings for 111 adults with acute head injury.

Case 4: Normal Pupils and Abnormal ABR in an Adult

A 21-year-old male was involved in a MVA, and sustained a severe head injury. Upon arrival of Life Flight, the patient was intubated while having grand mal seizures. Pupils were pinpoint and eyes were deviated to the right. Corneal and gag reflexes were intact. In the HHER, following helicopter transport, the patient still did not open eyes to painful stimuli and showed extensor posturing. GCS was 4. CT revealed multiple hemorrhagic contusions in the left frontal and temporal regions, the corpus callosum, and the right basal ganglia. A possible brainstem hemorrhage was noted, although artifact partially obscured the lower views. The perimesencephalic cistern was clearly defined.

The patient's ABR findings are illustrated and related to neurologic and physiologic findings in Figure 5-9. By post-injury day 2, increased ICP required barbiturate coma. Throughout the remaining days of the patient's hospital course, ICP was consistently less than 20 mmHg. However, on days 2 and 3,

there was a distinct prolongation in the wave I–III latency interval, the caudal brainstem transmission time. Brainstem neurologic signs were not valid, due to barbiturate therapy, but pupillary response was normal. On day 4, both ABR and pupillary findings were normal. The previously abnormal ABR, however, was an ominous indicator of possible brainstem dysfunction. Early on day 5, the caudal brainstem abnormality was again recorded. Within 3 hours, the ABR had deteriorated dramatically and the pupils were fixed and dilated bilaterally. Cerebral perfusion pressure appeared adequate (92 mmHg). Follow-up ABR assessment 2 hours later showed similarly abnormal findings. As these ABR abnormalities developed, we also observed a progressive increase in wave I amplitude. In the early morning of the sixth day, there was no ABR. Nuclear cerebral blood flow (CBF) studies indicated no cerebral circulation.

With this patient, ABR deterioration was repeatedly documented in the absence of any apparent pupillary abnormality. These changes seemed to predict impending overall neurologic decompensation and were perhaps electrophysiologic evidence of brainstem ischemia.

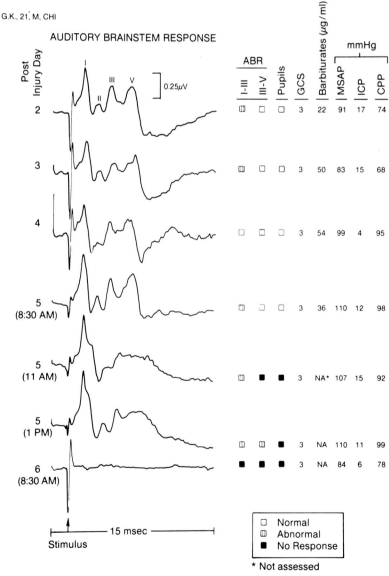

Figure 5-9. Serial auditory brainstem response (ABR) waveforms, neurologic and physiologic findings for 21-year-old male with severe closed head injury (Case 4). Note inconsistency in pupil and ABR data on several test dates.

Case 5: Abnormal Pupils and Normal ABR in an Adult

The patient was a 21-year-old female brought to the HHER by her mother because of a 2-day history of decreased mental status. When she was 11 months old, the patient had meningitis, and later placement of a ventriculo-peritoneal shunt. The history also included encephalitis at age 5 years. Since that time, the patient was treated with Dilantin for seizures. Upon hospital admission, the patient was lethargic but arousable by painful and verbal stimulation. Cranial nerve function was essentially intact, although pupils were 2 mm and very sluggishly reactive bilaterally. Bilateral Babinski reflexes were noted. Gait was normal except for some unsteadiness. A ventriculo-peritoneal shunt was inserted on the right on the 12th day post-admission. Subsequently, while the patient was still in the ICU, she remained stuporous and was not waking as expected. The right pupil was 4 mm and reactive, but the left pupil was 6 mm and fixed to light. Corneal reflexes were present. She localized to deep painful stimuli. A STAT CT scan was ordered, which showed normal ventricles, open cisterns, and no definite evidence of uncal herniation. Later on the day of surgery, the left pupil became fixed and dilated. Neurologic status was otherwise unchanged. ABRs were initially requested at this time. By the following day, the patient was opening her eyes to painful stimuli and vocalizing spontaneously (she had extubated herself). Pupillary responses were unchanged. GCS was 9 (eye, 3; motor, 5; verbal, 1). The next day, neurologic condition showed further improvement. The patient was following commands inconsistently. The pupillary abnormality on the left (cranial nerve III palsy) persisted. One week postoperatively, the patient was considerably improved, although she was dysarthric and disoriented with respect to time and place. She was discharged to home 1 month later with complete neurologic recovery, except for a residual left cranial nerve III palsy.

Serial ABR and AMR measurements were made on the day of surgery, the following 2 days, and then 1 week later (Fig. 5-10). A well-formed and reliable ABR was consistently recorded bilaterally. Brainstem transmission times were normal, and morphology of the rostral wave V component was excellent. The AMR was initially of small amplitude but repeatable and was observed at each test session to progressively increase in amplitude. On the basis of the neurophysiologic evidence of brainstem and cortical auditory integrity, the patient was not taken back to the OR for revision of the shunt, but, rather, closely monitored in the ICU even though the pupillary abnormality would have met traditional criteria for aggressive surgical management.

Case 6: Abnormal Pupils and Multimodality Evoked Responses

The patient was a 7-year-old male who suffered a closed head injury after being hit by a car while riding his bicycle. He was intubated and a placed on Pavulon upon arrival at the NWTH emergency receiving center. An emergency CT scan showed a small intracerebral hematoma in the right lateral occipital region surrounded by a small amount of edema. The CT scan also showed some subarachnoid blood on the right side of the tentorium and slight compression of the right lateral ventricle. Pupils were equal and reactive to light upon admission. On the second day, pupils were pinpoint for 1 hour, and on the third day they were sluggishly reactive for 15 hours. Then, over the next 2 days, the pupils returned to normal size and were equal and reactive to light. On the sixth post-injury day, the patient's pupils became fixed and dilated and remained that way for a week. At the end of this period, the pupils began to react sluggishly to light and the patient started to demonstrate decorticate posturing.

Evoked response testing was requested, after the pupils became fixed and dilated, because of concern about possible herniation. ABR test results were normal, demonstrating wave I–V latencies within the expected range bilaterally (Fig. 5-11). Although the ABR was normal, the other evoked response modalities yielded abnormal findings. There was no parietal component with median-nerve SSER recording and only slow diffuse activity seen with flash VER.

This patient's outcome has been poor. He was extubated and has regained consciousness, but has demonstrated poor motor performance. He has also had difficulty speaking. The application of multimodality evoked responses contributed to the intensive management. The clinical neurologic findings of persistently fixed and dilated pupils, in combination with absent SSERs, strongly suggested a severe CNS injury. The ABR, however, provided evidence of residual brainstem integrity and rationale for continued aggressive management.

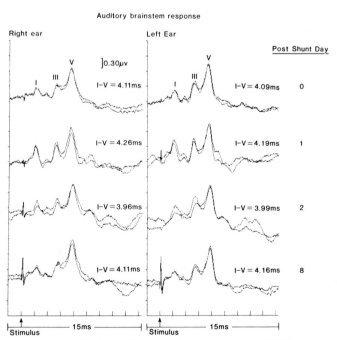

Figure 5-10. Serial auditory brainstem response (ABR) waveforms for a 21-year-old female with acute hydrocephalus and fixed and dilated pupils (Case 5).

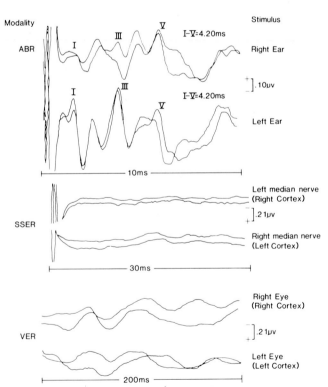

Figure 5-11. Auditory brainstem response (ABR), somatosensory evoked response (SSER), and visual evoked response (VER) waveforms for a 7-year-old male with severe head closed injury and fixed and dilated pupils at the time of testing (Case 6).

NEURORADIOLOGY

Current management of acute, severe brain injury is strongly dependent on neuroradiologic evidence of CNS structural status. The CT scan is especially crucial in clinical decision-making (Clifton et al., 1980; Fisher, 1984; French and Dublin, 1977; Narayan et al., 1981; Osborn, 1977; Rao et al., 1984; Teasdale et al., 1984; Toutant et al., 1984; Tsubokawa et al., 1980; Van Dongen et al., 1983; Zimmerman et al., 1978; Zuccarello et al., 1983). Other neuroradiologic techniques employed in brain injury include ultrasonography and nuclear cerebral blood flow (Goodman and Heck, 1977; Goodman et al., 1985). Relationships between AER findings and CT have been described by other investigators. Zuccarello et al. (1983) and Nagao et al. (1982) correlated brainstem lesions with CT and ABR. On the other hand, Tsubokawa et al. (1980) concluded that in comparing ABR findings with standard interpretation of CT, the ABR was the more valuable index of brainstem damage, particularly in patients for whom the CT suggested transtentorial herniation. Normal ABRs were recorded in patients with impending and even advanced CT evidence of herniation.

In collaboration with a neurosurgical colleague, Dr. Judy Mackey-Hargadine, we studied the association of ABR results (normal versus abnormal) and CT findings (neuroradiologist interpretation of transtentorial herniation versus no evidence of herniation). The results of this analysis were similar to the comparison of ABR and pupillary responses described above. Both relationships are illustrated in Figure 5-8. Although one might expect that a normal ABR would be found in patients with no evidence of transtentorial herniation and vice versa, there were many exceptions to this pattern. For example, over one-fifth of the patients with a "normal" CT scan, as defined by these criteria, had definite ABR abnormalities (usually wave I–V latency delays). Perhaps more surprising, a majority of the patients with

evidence of brainstem compression by CT yielded a normal ABR. Among this latter group were patients who survived the injury, as we will demonstrate with case reports to follow. Bedside ultrasonography is an important adjunct to CT, and a valuable means of daily neuroradiologic monitoring. The correlations among CT, ultrasound, and the ABR will also be highlighted by the cases. Perhaps, as Fisher (1984) suggested, the concepts underlying brain herniation need to be reassessed and the role of CT redefined.

Case 7: ABR, CT, and Ultrasound in an Adult

A 34-year-old male pedestrian was struck by an automobile and thrown a distance of 75 feet, sustaining a severe head injury. At the scene, he was hypotensive. Pupils were normally reactive on the right and sluggishly reactive on the left. GCS was 7. Ears were clear with no hemotympanum. Upon arrival at the HHER, pupils were 2 mm, round, and sluggishly reactive bilaterally. The patient was moving all extremities spontaneously. CT scan showed a left subdural hematoma and left subarachnoid blood, with a right-to-left midline shift and probable early transtentorial herniation (Fig. 5-12).

Serial ABRs (Fig. 5-13), CT scans, and ultrasound images (Fig. 5-14) were obtained over the course of the first month post-injury. On days 2 and 3, the neuroradiologist reported increased hemorrhage on the left, a progressive intracerebral hematoma in the left parietal-temporal region, increased midline shift, and definite transtentorial herniation. The perimesencephalic cistern was effaced, yet, the ABR during this period was normal and a poorly formed but reliable AMR was recorded (not shown). On the first ABR test date, pupils were 1 mm and unreactive, and inconsistencies between ABR, pupillary response and CT findings were repeatedly noted during the serially conducted assessments. In view of the worsening left-sided brain pathology and repeated episodes of increased ICP, a left temporal lobectomy (tip) was performed on the fifth day. Subsequent to this surgery, we continued to record AMR activity bilaterally. In addition, a normal ABR was recorded in the presence of pupillary abnormalities. This suggested residual brainstem integrity despite the early CT evidence of brainstem compression. The patient was transferred from the ICU to the neurosurgical floor.

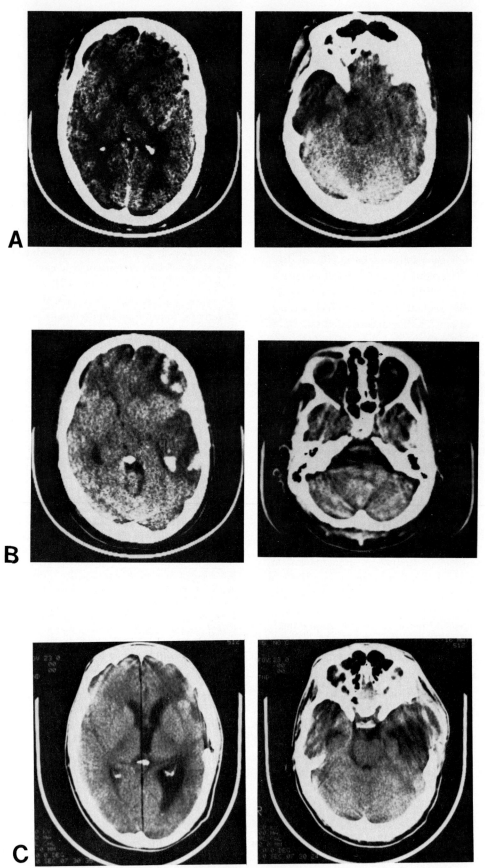

Figure 5-12. Serial computerized tomography (CT) scans for a 34-year-old male with closed head injury (Case 7). Initial scans on the day of injury (A) and again at post-injury day (B) showed evidence of transtentorial herniation. Final scans at day 30 (C) showed dilated ventricles.

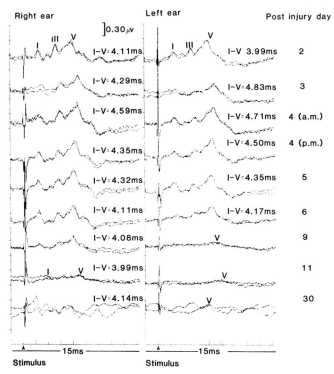

Auditory Brainstem Response

Right ear	Left ear	Post injury day
I–V=4.11ms	I–V 3.99ms	2
I–V=4.29ms	I–V=4.83ms	3
I–V=4.59ms	I–V=4.71ms	4 (a.m.)
I–V=4.35ms	I–V=4.50ms	4 (p.m.)
I–V=4.32ms	I–V=4.35ms	5
I–V=4.11ms	I–V=4.17ms	6
I–V=4.08ms		9
I–V=3.99ms		11
I–V=4.14ms		30

]0.30 μv

15ms
Stimulus

15ms
Stimulus

Figure 5-13. Serial auditory brainstem response (ABR) recordings for Case 7. ABR was initially normal.

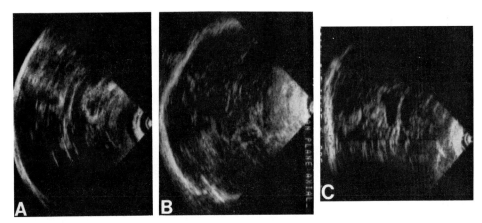

Figure 5-14. Serial ultrasonography through craniotomy for Case 7. Initial image shows left temporal hematoma. Final image shows dilated ventricles.

Case 8: Multimodality Evoked Responses and CT in a Child

The patient was a 4-year-old male who was involved in a motor vehicle accident. He was found unconscious at the scene and remained comatose during transport to the NWTH emergency receiving center. Physical examination revealed a linear laceration over the right and left posterior parietal occipital regions. Marked contusions were present across the forehead and both orbits. The right pupil was fixed and dilated and there was no movement of the right extremities. Initial CT scans during the acute phase showed a large left intracerebral hematoma, with edema compressing the left frontal and occipital horns (Fig. 5-15).

As seen in Figure 5-16, the ABR wave I–V intervals were normal bilaterally but the left-ear stimulus AMR was not observed. The VER waveforms were absent on the left cortex in response to flash stimulation to both eyes (Fig. 5-17). There was also no SSER left cortical component with median nerve stimulation. This multimodality evoked response pattern was repeated on follow-up evaluations. This case illustrates the increased precision of lesion localization and CT confirmation that is possible with the measurement of somatosensory and visual evoked response modalities in addition to the AERs.

APPLICATIONS OF AERs IN ACUTE BRAIN INJURY

MONITORING NEUROLOGIC STATUS WITH SERIAL RECORDINGS

As noted above, therapeutic modalities employed in the management of acute brain injury may invalidate the clinical neurologic examination. Sensory evoked potentials provide a noninvasive means of objectively evaluating CNS functional status over time, without contamination by necessary treatment regimens. Early reports of SERs in acute brain injury emphasized their possible value in predicting neurologic outcome (Greenberg and Becker, 1976; Greenberg et al., 1977). These pioneering studies generated the initial interest and excitement in the potential role of SERs in this challenging population. Prediction of both neurologic and cognitive/communicative outcome continues to be an important topic for clinical investigation. We have focused much of our effort on serially evaluating CNS function over time with SERs, rather than attempting to rely on data collected from a single test session 3 or 4 days after the injury, as other researchers have done (Anderson et al., 1984; Rappaport et al., 1978; Karnaze et al., 1982; Narayan et

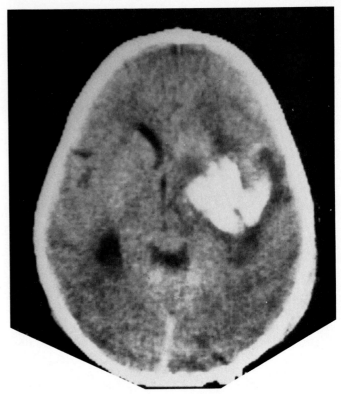

Figure 5-15. Computerized tomography for 4-year-old male with closed head injury (Case 8).

al., 1981; Lindsay et al., 1981; Rosenberg et al., 1984; Seales et al., 1979). As we will demonstrate below, serial evoked response data have varied applications in the acute period following severe brain injury. Maximum application of evoked responses is achieved when recordings are initially made within 24 hours of the injury and then repeated during the period of neurologic instability. We present evidence that the AMRs may be more useful in estimating quality of outcome than is the ABR. In previous reports (Hall and Mackey-Hargadine, 1984; Hall et al., 1985A,B; Hall and Tucker, 1985), we have stressed the point that an abnormal ABR almost always implied a poor out-

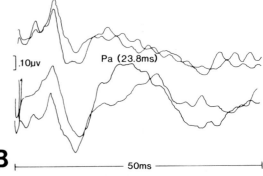

Figure 5-16. Auditory brainstem response (ABR) and auditory middle-latency response (AMR) waveforms for Case 8. A normal ABR was consistently recorded.

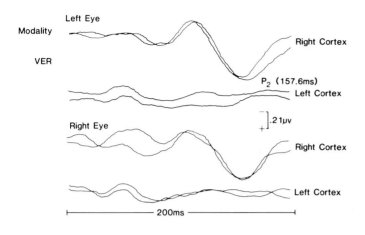

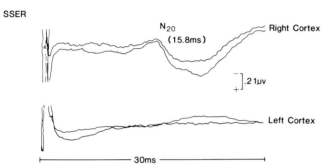

Figure 5-17. Somatosensory evoked responses and visual evoked responses for Case 8. Note absence of waveforms from left cortex for each modality.

come or death, whereas a normal acute ABR (within 24–76 hours post-injury) had little predictive value, and frequently was followed by patient death within the acute stage. This unfortunate sequence of events is related in many of the case reports in this chapter. Multimodality evoked responses, as we will show, often augment the clinical value of these serial measures.

Case 9: Neurologic Decompensation

A 30-year-old male exited a moving automobile and was then struck by another vehicle. He sustained a head injury and was transported via helicopter within 1 hour of the injury to the HHER. Upon arrival, pupils were 2 mm and non-reactive to light bilaterally. There were no oculocephalic reflexes and only a flicker motor response to deep painful stimuli. Corneal and gag reflexes were present. GCS was 4. Emergency CT showed cerebral contusions, severe diffuse edema on the left, and effacement of the perimesencephalic cistern. Following placement of an ICP monitor, he was transferred to the ICU, where initial AER assessment was carried out within 2 hours of the injury.

As depicted in Figure 5-18, an ABR, AMR, and apparent 40Hz response were recorded at this time. Brainstem transmission times for the ABR were within normal limits on the right but abnormally prolonged on the left. The AMR was of low amplitude but well-formed. Unfortunately, the patient developed serious ICP elevation that failed to respond to maximum medical therapy, including barbiturates. Over the initial 38 hours after the injury, there was a steady increase in ICP, presumably associated with cerebral vasomotor paralysis. As ICP increased, and cerebral perfusion pressure (CPP) decreased, we recorded a distinct rostral-caudal deterioration of the ABR (Fig. 5-19). The first change was an increase in the wave III–V latency, related in time to a decrease in CPP from the high 80s (mmHg) to the low 60s. With a reduction in CPP to below 30 mmHg, there was complete disappearance of wave V, and, over the course of less than an hour, changes in wave III morphology and latency. Only a large wave I and definite wave II component were observed with CPPs of less than 20 mmHg. Finally, with mean arterial pressure and ICP equivalent, the wave I component was no longer present. Nuclear cerebral perfusion could no longer be demonstrated on CBF studies.

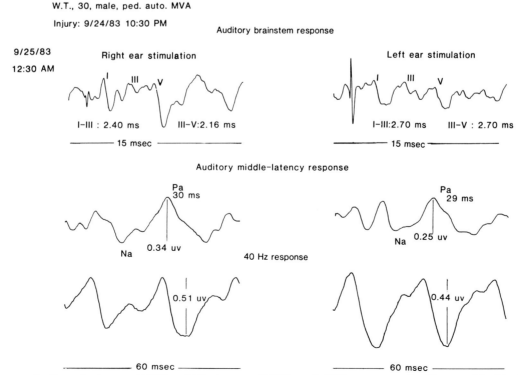

Figure 5-18. Auditory brainstem (ABR), middle-latency (AMR), and 40Hz responses for 30-year-old with closed head injury (Case 9). Data were obtained within 2 hours of the injury.

The preceding sequence of correlations among brain pathophysiology and the ABR all occured in the absence of detectable alterations in the clinical neurologic examination. The patient had persistently fixed and dilated pupils (from 18 hours onward) and no brainstem reflexes, perhaps due to barbiturate therapy. The case illustrates at least 4 features of serial ABR measurements in acute, severe brain injury: (1) Valid ABR data can be obtained within hours of the injury; (2) Early decisions on management of injury can be based, in part, on evoked response outcome. For example, the CT scan suggested transtentorial herniation and the neurologic examination yielded minimal responses, yet auditory brainstem and cortical (Celesia, 1976; Kaga et al., 1980; Lee et al., 1984)

responses were observed. Abnormal ABR findings on the left were probably a reflection of more intense brain swelling on the left, but evidence of residual brainstem integrity contributed to the decision to proceed very aggressively. High blood levels of alcohol may have suppressed CNS activity as reflected the clinical examination; (3) Significant changes in the ABR may document brainstem deterioration, even in the absence of detectable clinical changes in neurologic status; (4) With persistently elevated ICP, there are often rostral-caudal ABR abnormalities, presumably associated with brainstem ischemia (Hall et al., 1984A,B; Hall et al., 1985A,B; Hall and Tucker, 1985; Klug, 1982; McPherson et al., 1984; Mjoen et al., 1983; Newton et al., 1982; Nagao et al., 1979; Sato et al., 1984; Sohmer et al., 1982, 1983, 1984; Yagi & Baba, 1983).

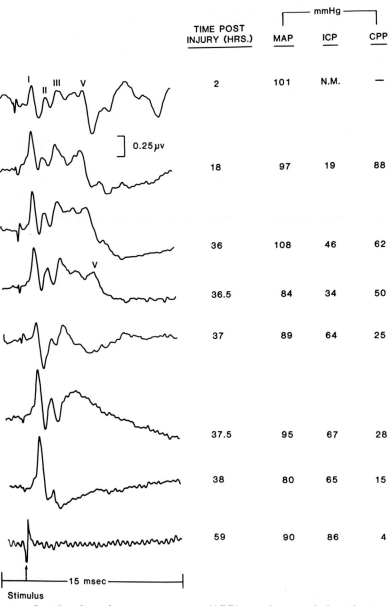

Figure 5-19.   Serial auditory brainstem response (ABR) waveforms and physiologic parameters for Case 9 during neurologic decompensation. Pupils were fixed and dilated after first test.

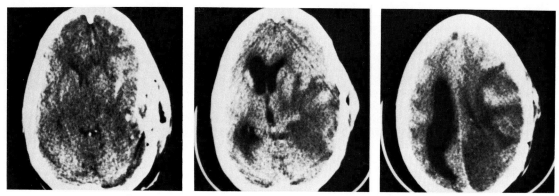

Figure 5-20. Computerized tomography for a 38-year-old male who was struck on the left temporal-parietal region of the head with a blunt object (Case 10).

Case 10: Surgical Intervention in a Head-Injured Adult

The patient was struck on the left temporal-parietal region with a blunt instrument. Upon arrival at the HHER, GCS was 6. Emergency CT (Fig. 5-20) showed evidence of a depressed skull fracture on the left and underlying large hemorrhagic intraparenchymal hematoma and edema with a mass effect creating a left-to-right midline shift. A mild degree of transtentorial herniation was also noted. Within the first 2 weeks post-injury, the patient's ICP became elevated, and following unsuccessful attempts to reduce it with traditional medical therapy, barbiturates were employed. A follow-up CT scan at 2 weeks revealed a left posterior cerebral artery infarct and persistent suggestion of transtentorial herniation (Fig. 5-20). ABR assessment was requested in light of these CT findings. As shown in Figure 5-21, the ABR wave III–V interpeak interval was markedly abnormal, although the caudal brainstem transmission time appeared to be within normal limits. The ABR suggested brainstem compression, providing neurophysiologic confirmation of the CT findings, and the patient was taken to the operating room for cerebral decompression. ICP monitored with a Richmond bolt at the time of ABR testing was 5 mmHg, a value that was considered spurious. An intraventricular catheter was inserted (opening pressure of 36 mmHg) and cerebral spinal fluid was drained. Upon return to the ICU, repeat ABR testing showed reversal of the wave III–V latency prolongation. Unfortunately, the next day ICP was persistently elevated despite regular CSF drainage, with a resultant decrease in CPP. An overall increase in brainstem transmission time was noted in the ABR. Twenty-four hours later, the ABR was very poorly formed. The patient was taken to the CT scanning area (Fig. 5-20), where he arrested and died.

The development of brainstem dysfunction and its reversal with aggressive therapy can be documented with the ABR. In combination, CT and the ABR offer strong evidence of CNS integrity or, conversely, compromise, and can therefore play a role in decisions regarding management. Other standard physiologic parameters (e.g., monitored ICP; Miller et al., 1984; Swann, 1984; Saul and Decker, 1982) may provide misleading information. The difficulties in clinical decision-making are, as we have stressed previously, compounded in patients in barbiturate coma.

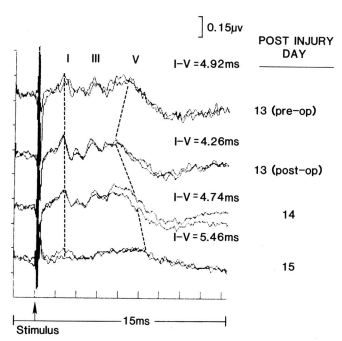

Figure 5-21. Serial auditory brainstem response (ABR) waveforms for Case 10 before and after surgical intervention.

Case 11: Surgical Intervention in a Child With Hydrocephalus

The patient was a 21-month-old male who came to the Texas Tech Health Science Center (TTHSC) ambulatory clinic with a history of hydrocephalus. Serial CT scans showed no significant changes in ventricular size, but the mother reported that the child was beginning to demonstrate signs of ataxia and irritability. Evoked response assessment yielded delayed flash VER waveforms of poor morphology and a mild delay in brainstem transmission times in the ABR (Figs. 5-22 and 5-23). The patient was admitted to the hospital and scheduled for surgery to insert a right ventriculo-peritoneal, low-pressure shunt. The neurosur-

geon reported that there was little CSF leakage when the dura was excised, a significant indicator for high-pressure status. Clear CSF under high pressure flowed well when a catheter was placed in the right lateral ventricle.

Repeat evoked response assessment 1 day after surgery revealed that the ABR I–V latencies had returned to normal and there were normal VER waveforms present over both occipital poles in response to flash stimulation (Figs. 5-22 and 5-23). The application of AERs and VERs in hydrocephalus have been reported by others (Guthkelch et al., 1982; Kraus et al., 1984; Sklar et al., 1979; York et al., 1981). In the present case report, ABR and VER results reflected increased ICP not shown by the CT scan and documented the return of normal neural conduction after surgical intervention.

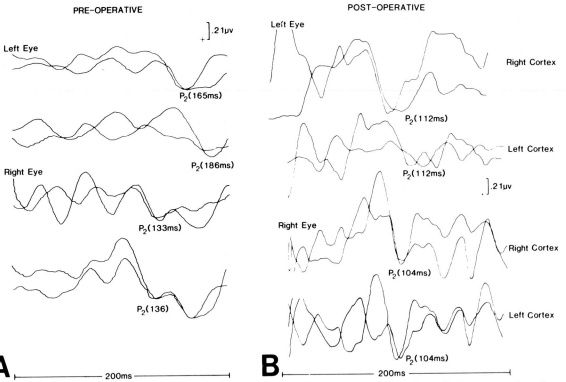

Figure 5-22. Visual evoked response (VER) waveforms before and after ventriculo-peritoneal shunt procedure for a 21-month-old male with acute hydrocephalus (Case 11).

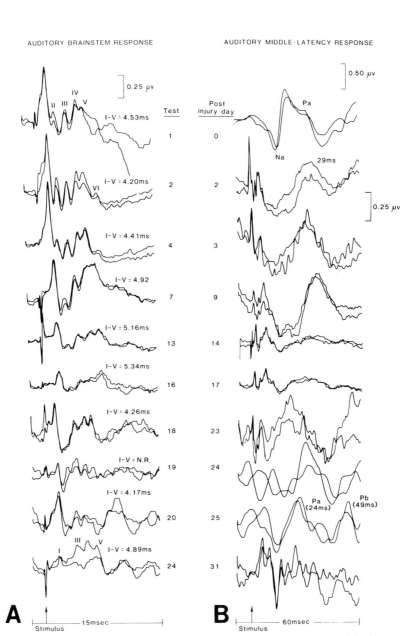

AUDITORY BRAINSTEM RESPONSE   AUDITORY MIDDLE-LATENCY RESPONSE

Figure 5-23. Serial auditory brainstem response (ABR) and auditory middle-latency response (AMR) waveforms for a 22-year-old male with closed head injury (Case 12). Changes in ABR were associated with medical management of hypotension.

Case 12: Medical Management in a Head-Injured Adult

A 22-year-old male suffered a head injury in a MVA. At the scene, pupils were sluggishly reactive and respirations were labored. There was a decorticate motor response. GCS was 5. Following helicopter transport to HHER and emergency therapy en route, pupils were equal and briskly reactive to light. Motor responses were purposeful to deep painful stimuli, but there was still no eye opening or verbal response. Emergency CT showed a right intraventricular bleed and a small left subdural hematoma. He was taken to the OR for a ventriculostomy (opening pressure was 12 cm H_2O) and then to the ICU.

A chronologic summary of this patient's physiologic status during the first month after the injury is displayed in Table 5-2. For the initial 3 days, ICP was controlled with frequent doses of hyperosmolar (mannitol) drugs, as well as hyperventilation and CSF drainage. By one week, however, ICP was increasing to the 40s (mmHg) and barbiturate therapy was instituted. The major medical problem during barbiturate coma was a series of episodes of hypotension that were treated with dopamine. Follow-up CT scans indicated resolution of the intraventricular hemorrhage, and neurologic status began to improve. Over the course of the next 2 weeks, the patient developed adult respiratory distress syndrome, at one point requiring cardiopulmonary resuscitation (CPR). He arrested and died 1 month after the injury.

Serial AER measures in this patient are illustrated in Figures 5-23 and 5-24. There were repeated instances of abnormalities in brainstem times, persisting for almost a week at one period, which were reversed coincident with pharmacologic elevation of mean arterial pressure. On day 19, a wave V component was not observed with the standard electrode array (Fig. 5-23), but evaluation of the ABR with a four-channel recording array revealed a repeatable wave V (Fig. 5-24). The AMR, in contrast, was relatively stable although suppressed, of course, during barbiturate coma. Finally, within 24 hours of the patient's death, ABR abnormalities were again recorded, this time in conjunction with no apparent AMR. The pathophysiologic feature associated temporally with the

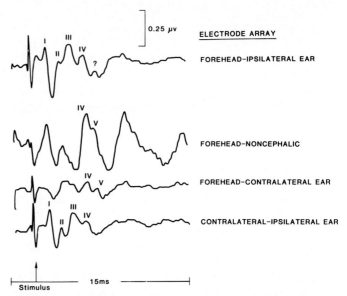

Figure 5-24. Simultaneous four-channel auditory brainstem response recordings for Case 12 on day 19. Note apparent absence of wave V component with traditional electrode array, but presence on alternative array.

ABR changes was reduced CPP, resulting not from elevated ICP but, rather, from decreased MAP. On the basis of the ABR findings, it would appear that CPPs in the 60s (mmHg) were inadequate for maintaining normal brainstem function of an already damaged CNS. An additional factor to consider, at least on day 14, was hypoxia. Repeated hypoxic episodes toward the end of the patient's hospital course may have also contributed to the terminal ABR abnormalities.

Table 5-2 Chronologic Summary of Physiologic Parameters for 22-Year-Old-Male with Severe Closed Head Injury (Case 12). See Figures 23 and 24 for Auditory Evoked Response Findings.

Test Number	Post Injury day	Temperature (°C)	MAP	ICP	CPP	PaO₂	PaCO2*	Medications†			
			(mmHg)					Morph.	Meto.	Mann.	Barb.
1	0	38.2	103	8	95	128	28	−	+	+	−
2	2	38.1	81	15	66	127	23	+	+	+	−
4	4	38.6	88	21	67	225	25	+	+	+	−
7	9	35.0	119	9	110	142	23	+	+	+	−
13	14	35.6	77	8	69	64	35	−	−	−	40 μg/ml
16	17	34.9	68	10	58	125	26	−	−	−	70 μg/ml
18	23	38.5	90	NM	CNE	90	30	−	−	−	−
19	24	38.4	81	NM	CNE	73	33	−	−	−	−
20	25	38.3	83	NM	CNE	75	36	−	−	−	−
24	31	39.2	87	NM	CNE	95	50	−	−	−	−

* MAP = mean arterial pressure; ICP = intracranial pressure; CPP = cerebral perfusion pressure; PaO₂ = arterial pressure oxygen; PaCO₂ = arterial pressure carbon dioxide.

† morphine, metocurine, mannitol, barbiturates; + = administered within four hours preceding auditory evoked response testing; NM = not monitored; CNE = could not evaluate.

DEFINING BRAIN DEATH

Diagnosis of brain death is based on evidence of cerebral and brainstem neuronal inactivity (Korein, 1980). There are numerous criteria for definition of brain death, and considerable medical, legal, and ethical discussion of the topic (Beresford, 1984; Guidelines, 1981). The primary mode of assessment in the determination of brain death has been and will be the neurological examination. Current therapeutic modalities in acute, severe brain injury, as we have already pointed out, may compromise the validity of the neurologic examination. Also, in the era of organ transplantation, some of the criteria that require an established time period of physiologic inactivity before brain death can be declared are simply not feasible, since they preclude obtaining viable organs. We have, therefore, evaluated the usefulness of SERs as ancillary procedures in the diagnosis of brain death.

In collaboration with colleagues in neurosurgery and neuroradiology (Drs. J. Mackey-Hargadine and E. Kim of the University of Texas Medical School, Houston), we have recently reported group data and case reports in support of this timely application of SERs. These papers have been limited to experience in adult brain-injured populations (Hall and Mackey-Hargadine, 1985; Hall et al., 1985B; Hall and Tucker, 1985). We have found a strong correlation between the ABR and nuclear cerebral blood flow (CBF) measures (Goodman and Heck, 1977; Goodman et al., 1985) in over 80 adults with acute severe brain injury. The majority of these patients were chemically paralyzed or in barbiturate coma at the time of assessment, and some were evaluated within the first 6 hours after injury with recreational drugs in the blood.

The relationship between ABR and nuclear CBF for a group of 50 patients with traumatic head injury is illustrated in Figure 5-25. Eliminated from this analysis are patients with acute cerebral vascular accidents. All of the patients with normal CBF had either a normal ABR or at least wave components I and III. None of the patients without CBF had an ABR. In this group, most patients had no response, while one-third had a wave I and no

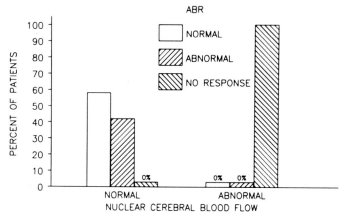

Figure 5-25. Relationship of auditory brainstem response (ABR) and nuclear cerebral blood flow (CBF) for 50 patients with traumatic head injury.

other components. Thus, in traumatic head injury, the ABR versus CBF relationship is very strong and statistically significant (at .000001 level of confidence).

Case 13: ABR and CBF in Determining Brain Death in an Adult

A 24-year-old male sustained a gunshot wound to the right temporal region. The patient was transferred to the HHER with normal vital signs but minimal neurologic function. Pupils were midposition and unreactive. GCS was 5. Blood alcohol level was 158 mg/dl. He was taken to CT scanning, which showed a right subdural hematoma, and then directly to the OR for a right temporal craniotomy and evacuation of the hematoma, with ventriculostomy. Marked brain swelling was noted intraoperatively. This was treated with hyperventilation, diuretics, and barbiturates with little success. Postoperatively, the patient did poorly, and required Dopamine for support of blood pressure. By the evening of the injury, there was no evidence of cerebral activity by clinical examination. There was no movement to deep pain. Pupils were fixed in midposition. Brainstem reflexes were absent. Apnea response was not assessed in the face of barbiturates.

Initial AER assessment was carried out at this time. As illustrated in Figure 5-26, a well-formed ABR was recorded from the left. No response could be generated with right-ear stimulation at maximum intensity levels. There was no AMR bilaterally but this finding was considered equivocal due the barbiturate therapy. Nuclear CBF studies were requested. The image on the left portion of Figure 5-27 indicates that flow was present. On the following morning, ABR assessment was again carried out. Neurologic status, examined after chemical paralysis was medically reversed, showed no brainstem or cerebral signs except for minimal right corneal reflex. Once again a normal ABR was recorded. ICP continued to increase into the mid 30s (mmHg) in spite of maximum medical therapy. Repeat ABRs later on day 1 after the injury yielded no response. A second nuclear CBF study failed to document flow and the patient was declared brain dead. The patient was promptly taken to the OR for a donor nephrectomy and splenectomy. Two normal kidneys were donated.

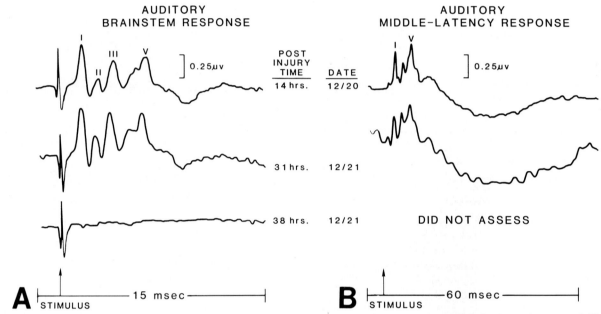

Figure 5-26.   Serial auditory brainstem response (ABR) waveforms for a 24-year-old male with fatal gunshot wound (Case 13).

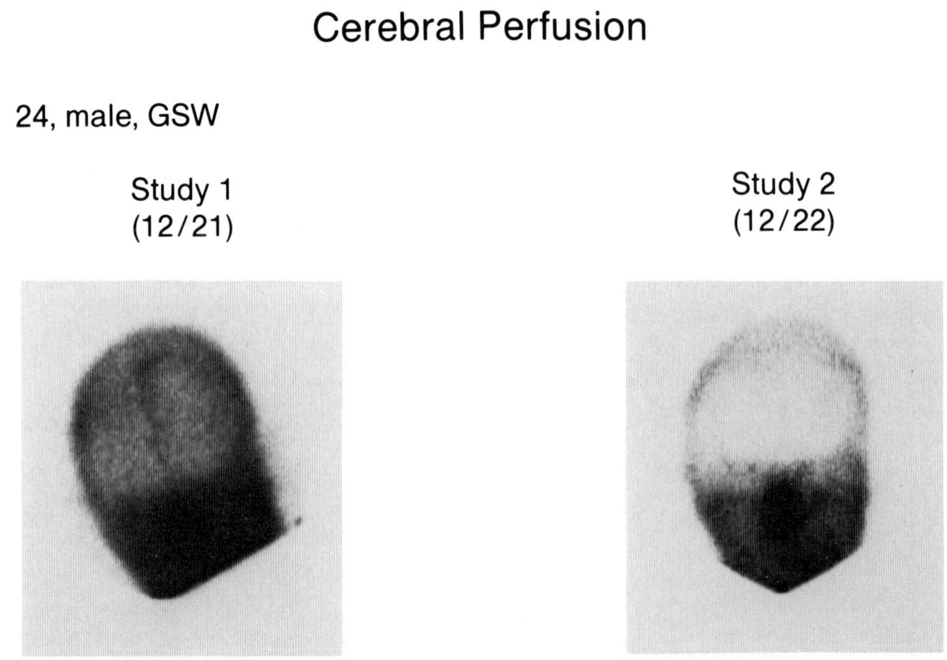

Cerebral Perfusion

24, male, GSW

Study 1
(12/21)

Study 2
(12/22)

Figure 5-27.   Two nuclear cerebral blood flow studies for Case 13. See Figure 5-26 for ABR findings on test days.

Case 14: Adult Determination of Brain Death

The patient was a 43-year-old involved in a MVA who sustained multiple injuries, including chest injury, severe facial trauma, and head injury. She was hypotensive at the scene and required CPR. GCS was 3 when Life Flight transported the patient to the HHER. Neurologic status improved with aggressive emergency therapy. GCS was 7. However, following CT scanning, which showed diffuse brain swelling, and transfer to the ICU, GCS was again 3. Pupils were 2 mm and unreactive. There were no brainstem reflexes. The patient was flaccid.

The organ transplantation team was notified of the patient's condition.

AERs were first recorded within 12 hours after the injury with the patient's status as described above. As seen in Figure 5-28, there was a normal ABR bilaterally, although only right-ear stimulus data are shown, but no apparent AMR. This finding provided further rationale for aggressive medical therapy. The following day, an ABR was again recorded with all brainstem transmission times within normal limits and a reliable AMR was observed. Additional testing on post-injury day 6 confirmed these findings. After a hospital course of 6 weeks, the patient was discharged to home. Followup AER assessment 9 months later continue to show normal brainstem and cortical auditory functioning.

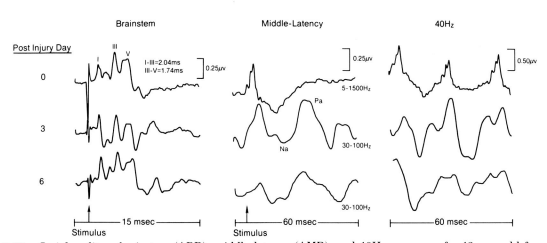

Figure 5-28.   Serial auditory brainstem (ABR), middle-latency (AMR), and 40Hz responses for 43-year-old female with multiple trauma, including head injury (Case 14) evaluated for brain death.

Case 15: Pediatric Confirmation of Brain Death

The patient was an 11-year-old male who was brought to the emergency room after nearly drowning at a local swimming pool. He was found apneic and without a detectable pulse. CPR was initiated by paramedics at the scene. Upon arrival at the hospital, he was hypotensive and hypothermic. He was given Dopamine and placed on a heating blanket. Controlled hyperventilation was begun in order to decrease ICP. A neurologic examination revealed no gag reflex, no corneal reflexes, and no response to a cold-water caloric stimulus (oculovestibular reflex). No cough could be elicited. The patient was unresponsive to deep, painful stimuli.

An EEG was obtained that showed a markedly depressed background of nearly unreadable electrical activity. Diagnosis was profound anoxic encephalopathy with nearly complete loss of brainstem and cerebral hemisphere function. Evoked response assessment was carried out one hour after admission (Fig. 5-29). Initial VER tests showed some early activity, but no cortical components were observed. Only ABR waves I and III were observed on initial assessment, indicating severe rostral brainstem pathology. Repeat tests failed to demonstrate significant improvement. The patient expired after being removed from the ventilator 24 hours later. As noted above, evoked responses may contribute to the determination of brain death in adults. This case illustrates an application of two modality evoked responses in defining brain death in a child. The VERs and neurologic examination suggested brainstem and cortical inactivity. The presence of an ABR wave III, however, indicated residual brainstem function and was not compatible with brain death. Based on our experiences, such a marked ABR abnormality is strongly associated with poor neurologic outcome, usually death. This neurophysiologic information is useful in counseling the family regarding patient prognosis.

Case 16: Pediatric Determination of Brain Death

The patient was a 15-month-old female who initially presented to a local community hospital with a 1-week history of high fever. A spinal tap was done and a diagnosis of *Hemophilus influenzae* meningitis was made. She was transferred to a regional hospital pediatric ICU. Shortly after admission, the patient had generalized grand mal seizures lasting 3–7 minutes. She was started on phenobarbital and antibiotic therapy. Several hours later, her pupils were unreactive and she began to demonstrate decerebrate posturing. She was paralyzed with Pavulon and was intubated, and controlled hyperventilation was initiated. Emergency CT scan revealed marked hydrocephalus.

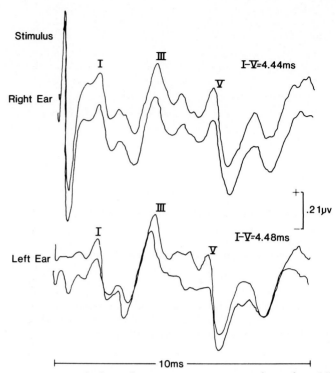

Figure 5-30. Auditory brainstem response waveforms for a 15-month-old female with meningitis with minimal neurologic signs evaluated for brain death (Case 16).

After 2 days of hospitalization, the attending physician suspected brain death and requested an ABR assessment. The initial ABR showed a well-formed response with a mild delay in the neural conduction time between waves I and V (Fig. 5-30). Because of the results of the ABR testing, the physician decided to continue aggressive treatment for increased ICP. A repeat ABR obtained 2 days later indicated no change in waveform latencies or amplitude. The patient was later successfully extubated. Unfortunately, she did not regain consciousness, and as of this writing continues to exhibit severe neurological deficits.

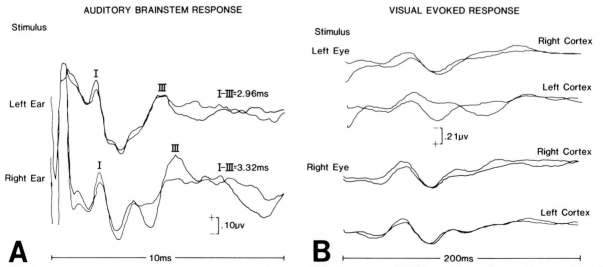

Figure 5-29. Auditory brainstem response (ABR) and visual evoked response (VER) waveforms for an 11-year-old male drowning victim evaluated for determination of brain death (Case 15).

PREDICTING COGNITIVE/COMMUNICATIVE OUTCOME

As noted in the introduction of this chapter, estimation of long-term outcome was the objective of the earliest studies of SERs in severe head injury (Greenberg and Becker, 1976; Greenberg et al., 1977). These important clinical reports provided the motivation for our research and applications of AERs in this challenging population and have led to ongoing interest and clinical research by others (Anderson et al., 1984; Greenberg et al., 1981; Karnaze et al., 1982; Narayan et al., 1981; Newton et al., 1982; Rappaport et al., 1978; Rosenberg et al., 1984; Seales et al., 1979). Without exception, these previously reported studies have based estimates of long-term outcome on SER data acquired typically during a single test session subsequent to the third day post-injury.

We have studied the relationship between serial AER data obtained within the first week after injury and cognitive/communicative outcome at 3 months as described with the Ranchos Los Amigos Hospital Scale (RLAHS) (Hagen et al., 1984) in 74 survivors of severe head injury. None were in barbiturate coma at the time of testing. Mean GCS was 5.7. Data for patients dying within the first post-injury week were not analyzed. The results are displayed in Figure 5-31. Patients with excellent recovery (RLAHS VIII) invariably had a consistently normal AMR during the first week post-injury. All but 5 percent of the patients with good recovery (RLAHS VII), and 19 percent of those with fair recovery (RLAHS IV–V), also yielded normal AMRs in the acute period. Among the patients with poor recovery (RLAHS I–IV), a majority had either an abnormal response (low amplitude) or no AMR within the first week after injury. While these findings are only preliminary, they do appear to suggest that a complete recovery depends on integrity of the neuroanatomic region generating the AMR, perhaps primary auditory cortex (Celesia, 1976; Kaga et al., 1980; Lee et al., 1984).

Not unexpectedly, some 32 percent of the patients with a very unfavorable outcome, at least at 3 months after the injury, had normal AMRs bilaterally. Other neuroanatomic regions are, of course, vital for normal speech/language/cognitive functioning, regions other than just the primary auditory cortex, and these regions may have sustained substantial damage. In addition, it is likely that in many cases significant further cognitive/communicative improvement occurred after the month limit of this study. We plan to follow this patient series for a full year post-injury and to increase the number of subjects. A promising new area for research on predicting long-term cognitive outcome in head injury is exploitation of the auditory P 300 (P3) response, a true cognitive neurophysiologic event (Levin, 1985).

Case 17: Normal AMRs and Good Outcome

A 19-year-old male, involved in a MVA, was admitted to the HHER with a GCS of 7. CT showed diffuse cerebral swelling and blood in the right portion of the perimesencephalic cistern. Opening ICP on insertion of a monitoring device was 14 cmH₂O. ICP during the acute phase was managed adequately with maximum medical therapy. Serial AMRs were measured during this time period (Fig. 5-32). Throughout the first 19 days after injury, we consistently recorded a normal AMR and a normal ABR (not shown). At 3 months, the patient was

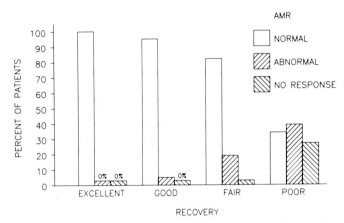

Figure 5-31. Relationship between serial acute auditory middle-latency response (AMR) and cognitive/communicative outcome at 3 months post-injury in 74 survivors of head injury.

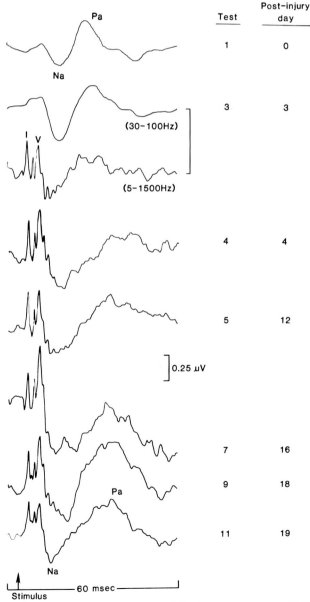

Figure 5-32. Serial auditory middle-latency response (AMR) waveforms for a 19-year-old male with severe closed head injury and good recovery (Case 17).

following commands. He was oriented and exhibited awareness of self, body, family, and environment. Judgement and insight were reduced but improving. RLAHS was VII.

Case 18: Abnormal AMRs and Poor Outcome

A 28-year-old male sustained a head injury when the automobile he was driving struck a tree. He was admitted to the HHER with a GCS of 4. CT showed diffuse cerebral edema with no discrete intracranial mass lessions. An ICP monitor was placed in the OR. Opening pressure was 7 cmH₂O. ICP was con-

trolled with medical therapy. Within 2 days, only chemical paralysis and sedation were required to maintain normal ICP. Three weeks post-injury, best GCS was 10 and there was a persistent left hemiparesis.

Serial AMR findings are shown in Figure 5-33. At 8 hours post-injury, there appeared to be a poorly formed, low-amplitude Pa wave component of the AMR when the response was recorded with a limited filter setting (30–100Hz), but not with a wide setting (5–1500Hz), which we customarily use if muscle artifact is not excessive. In subsequent recordings through day 20, we did not observe a reliable, clearly-defined AMR Pa component. Three months post-injury, the patient's RLAHS was III. He opened his eyes to commands and visually attended, but inconsistently followed simple commands.

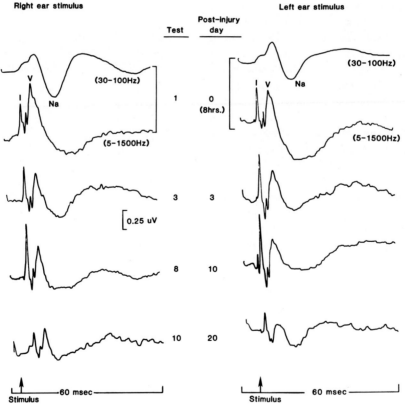

Figure 5-33.   Serial auditory middle-latency response (AMR) waveforms for a 28-year-old male with severe closed head injury and poor recovery (Case 18).

Case 19: Multimodality Responses and Outcome; Predicting Cognitive/Communicative Outcome with SER and VERs

The patient was a 12-year-old male who received a gunshot wound to the head while hunting. He was comatose upon arrival at the emergency room. An emergency CT scan showed a bullet track through left frontal, temporal, and occipital lobes. There was a fracture in the left occipital area and bone fragments were present in the left occiput. An emergency craniotomy and decompression were performed and a pressure bandage was placed around the head. The child was admitted to the pediatric ICU and was given medical therapy to decrease ICP.

Immediately after surgery, ABRs were carried out to evaluate brainstem function. Normal waveforms were present bilaterally and neural conduction times between wave I and wave V were within normal limits (Fig. 5-34). When the pressure bandage was removed the next day, VER and SER testing was done. VERs were clearly present in the right occipital derivation; however, no VER waveforms were recorded from the left occipital derivation. SER median nerve recordings showed a very small amplitude right parietal component. Responses were not observed from the left parietal cortex (Fig. 5-34). In this case, the VER and SER demonstrated a localized lesion in the left cerebral hemisphere, though the ABR was normal bilaterally.

The child was successfully extubated and later transferred to a rehabilitation center for speech, physical, and occupational therapies. The speech pathologist reports the child demonstrated telegraphic speech when he began therapy and there was an asymmetry in the right facial muscle tone and control. During therapy, his verbal expression improved from telegraphic speech to communication characterized by word-finding difficulty, circumlocutions, disruptive communication, and a reduction of length and completeness of sentences. His reading and writing abilities were severely limited. His final diagnosis was aphasia compatible with generalized brain damage. The absence of VER and SER waveforms on the left side served as a good prognostic indicator of speech and language outcome.

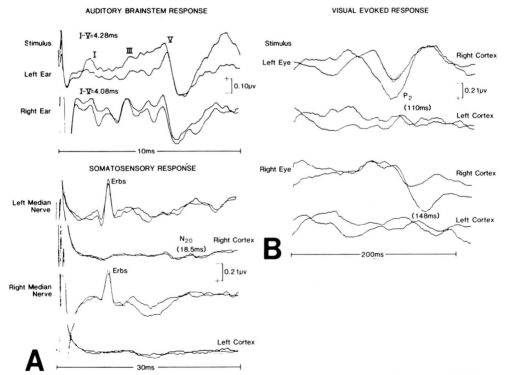

Figure 5-34. Auditory brainstem response (ABR), somatosensory evoked response (SSER), and visual evoked response (VER) waveforms for a 12-year-old male with a gunshot wound. Two months post-injury, patient had residual aphasia. Note normal ABR but marked SSER abnormality (Case 19).

CONCLUSION

SER recordings from comatose, severely brain-injured children and adults are clinically feasible and contribute in varied ways to acute medical and surgical management. Serial SER measurements are particularly useful. There are currently in our experience at least 6 main applications of SERs in this challenging population.

1. Monitoring neurologic status, especially in patients whose medical therapy or depth of coma limits the information gained from the clinical neurologic examination.
2. Localizing CNS dysfunction and functional correlation of neuroradiologic findings.
3. Documentation of the effects of medical and/or surgical therapy on CNS status.
4. Confirmation of the information gained from traditional measures of CNS status in acute injuries, such as the neurologic examination, physiologic monitors (e.g., MAP, ICP, CPP).
5. Determination of brain death.
6. Prediction of long-term neurologic outcome, including quality of survival.

In this chapter, we have attempted to summarize our clinical experiences with SER measurement of over 900 brain-injured patients. Based on these experiences, we are excited about the unique role SERs can play in rational, aggressive, and effective management of brain injury. However, we hasten to acknowledge the paucity of current basic understanding of the relationship among SERs and the pathophysiology of brain injury, and among SERs and other neurodiagnostic measures. There is mounting evidence linking alterations in SERs with brain ischemia. An important need exists for experimental and clinical studies to define the correlation between specific types of SER changes (e.g., latency versus amplitude) and the stage of the ischemic process, and also the portion of the CNS involved (e.g., brainstem versus cerebrum, and white matter versus gray matter). Such investigation is now underway (Astrup et al., 1977; Astrup, 1982; Benegin et al., 1981; Goitein et al., 1983A,B; Hargadine et al., 1980; Heiss & Rosner, 1983; Hossman & Kleihues, 1973; Lesnick et al., 1984; Lutschg et al., 1983; Nakagawa et al., 1984; Sohmer et al., 1983; Umbach et al., 1981; Stern et al., 1982; Sutton et al., 1980).

There are a number of promising avenues for future clinical research. Increased automation of SER recording is an advantage for continuous monitoring and cost containment. Trials are needed to evaluate the feasibility of this concept in the ICU. The relationships among types and severity of brain injury, acute management, SERs, and neurologic outcome probably differ for children versus adults (Bruce et al., 1978; Shapiro, 1985). To date, much of the above-noted research has been conducted with adult populations. Comparisons of these relations in an adequate series of pediatric versus adult patients, with carefully described brain pathologies, would be very useful clinically. Finally, prediction of the quality of survival and neurophysiologic correlation of degree of residual brain dysfunction, and even potential for further recovery, is of ongoing theoretical and clinical interest. The brainstem SERs appear to be inadequate for this application. The cortical components of multimodality evoked responses, especially the cognitive (P 300 or P3)

responses, may be extremely useful in this regard (Levin, 1985). In closing, we are encouraged by the cumulative clinical experiences with SERs in acute brain injury that have been reported during the past decade and foresee an even greater experimental and clinical research effort in the coming years.

ACKNOWLEDGMENTS

We gratefully acknowledge the invaluable support of Drs. Judy Mackey-Hargadine and Steven Fletcher, Division of Neurosurgery, and Dr. Nabil F. Maklad, Department of Radiology, University of Texas Medical School/Hermann Hospital, Houston; and of Drs. Rolf Habersang, Marita Angleton, and Peter Bickers, Department of Pediatrics; and of Drs. Jeffrey Cone and Wayne Paullus, Department of Neurosurgery, Texas Tech Health Science Center/Northwest Texas Hospital, Amarillo. This work was supported in part by the 1985 Braintree Hospital Award for Outstanding Research in Head Injury (received by Dr. Hall).

REFERENCES

Aguilar, EA III, Hall, JW III, Mackey-Hargadine, JR (1986). Neuro-otologic evaluation of the acute severely head-injured patient: Correlation among physical findings, auditory evoked responses and computerized tomography. *Otolaryngol Head Neck Surg*, 94, 211–219 in press

Anderson, DC, Bundlie, S, Rockswold, GL (1984). Multimodality evoked potentials in closed head trauma. *Arch Neurol*, 41, 369–374

Astrup, J, Symon, L, Branston, NM, Lassen, NA (1977). Cortical evoked potential and extracellular K+ and H+ at critical levels of brain ischemia. *Stroke*, 8, 51–57

Astrup, J (1982). Energy-requiring cell functions in the ischemic brain: Their critical supply and possible inhibition in protective therapy. *J Neurosurg*, 56, 482–497

Beresford, HR (1984). Legal aspects of terminating care. *Semin Neurol*, 4, 23–29

Bruce, DA, Shut, L, Bruno, LA, Wood, JH, Sutton, LN (1978). Outcome following severe head injuries in children. *J Neurosurg*, 48, 679–688

Bunegin, L, Ablin, MA, Helsel, P, Herrera, R (1981). Cerebral blood flow and evoked response. *J Cereb Blood Flow Metab*, 1 (Suppl. 1), s226–s227

Celesia, GG (1976). Organization of auditory cortical areas in man. *Brain*, 15, 465–482

Clifton, GL, Grossman, RG, Makela, ME, et al. (1980). Neurological course and correlated computerized tomography findings after severe closed head injury. *J Neurosurg*, 52, 611–624

Fisher, CM (1984). Acute brain herniation: A revised concept. *Sem Neurol*, 4, 417–421

French, BN, Dublin, AB (1977). The value of computerised tomography in 1000 consecutive head injuries. *Surg Neurol*, 7, 171–183

Goitein, KJ, Amit, Y, Fainmesser, P, Sohmer, H (1983B). Diagnostic and prognostic value of auditory nerve brainstem evoked responses in comatose children. *Crit Care Med*, 11, 91–94

Goitein, K, Fainmesser, P, Sohmer, H (1983A). Cerebral perfusion pressure and auditory brain-stem responses in childhood CNS diseases. *Am J Dis Child*, 137, 777–781

Goodman, JM, Heck, LL (1977). Confirmation of brain death at bedside by isotope angiography. *JAMA*, 238, 966–968

Goodman, JM, Heck, LL, Moore, BD (1985). Confirmation of brain death with portable isotope angiography: A review of 204 cases. *Neurosurgery*, 16, 492–497

Greenberg, RP, Becker, DP (1976). Clinical applications and results of evoked potential data in patients with severe head injury. *Surgical Forum*, 26, 484–486

Greenberg, RP, Becker, DP, Miller, JD, Mayer, DJ (1977). Evaluation of brain function in severe head trauma with multi-modality evoked potentials. Part II. Localization of brain dysfunction in correlation with post-traumatic neurologic condition. *J Neurosurg, 47*, 163–177

Greenberg, RP, Newlon, PG, Hyatt, MS, Narayan, RD, Becker, DP (1981). Prognostic implication of early multimodality evoked potentials in severely head-injured patients. A prospective study. *J Neurosurg, 55*, 227–236

Guidelines for the determination of death (1981). Report of the medical consultants on the diagnosis of death to the President's commission for the study of ethical problems in medicine and biomedical and behavioral research. Special communication. *JAMA, 246*, 2184–2186

Guthkelch, AN, Sclabassi, RJ, Vries, JK (1982). Changes in the visual evoked potentials of hydrocephalic children. *Neurosurgery, 11*, 599–602

Hagen, C, Malkmus, D, Durham, P (1984). *The levels of cognitive functioning scale.* Professional Staff Association, Ranchos Los Amigos Hospital, Downey, CA

Hall, JW III, Huangfu, M, Gennarelli, TA (1982). Auditory function in acute severe head injury. *Laryngoscope, 92*, 883–890

Hall, JW III, Huangfu, M, Gennarelli, TA, et al. (1983A). Auditory evoked responses, impedance measures and diagnostic speech audiometry in severe head injury. *Otolaryngol Head Neck Surg, 91*, 50–60

Hall, JW III, Huangfu, M, Gennarelli, TA, et al. (1983B). Auditory brainstem abnormalities in experimental and clinical acute severe head injury. *Trans Pa Acad Ophthalmol Otolaryngol, 36*, 86–88

Hall, JW III, Brown, DP, Mackey-Hargadine, JR (1984A). Pediatric applications of serial auditory brainstem and middle-latency evoked response recordings. *Int J Pediatr Otorhinolaryngol, 9*, 201–218

Hall, JW III, Mackey-Hargadine, JR (1984). Auditory evoked responses in severe head injury. *Semin Hear, 5*, 313–336

Hall, JW III, Morgan, SH, Mackey-Hargadine, JR, et al. (1984B). Neuro-otologic applications of simultaneous multi-channel auditory evoked response recordings. *Laryngoscope, 94*, 883–889

Hall, JW III (1985). Effects of high-dose barbiturates on acoustic reflexes and auditory evoked responses. *Acta Otolaryngol, 100*, 387–398

Hall, JW III, Mackey-Hargadine, JR (1986). Sensory evoked potentials in the diagnosis of brain death. In ME Miner & K Wagner (Eds.), *Neurotrauma: Treatment, Rehabilitation and Related Issues.* Butterworths: Stoneham, MA. pp. 133–153

Hall, JW III, Mackey-Hargadine, JR, Allen, SJ (1985A). Monitoring neurologic status of comatose patients in the intensive care unit. In JJ Jacobson (Eds.), *Auditory brain-stem response* (pp. 253–283). San Diego: College Hill Press

Hall, JW III, Mackey-Hargadine, JR, Kim, EE (1985B). Auditory brainstem response (ABR) in determination of brain death. *Arch Otolaryngol, 111*, 613–620

Hall, JW III, Tucker, DA (1985). Auditory evoked responses in traumatic head injury. *The Hearing J, 38*, 23–29

Hall, JW III, Tucker, DA (1986). Sensory evoked responses in the intensive care unit. *Ear Hear, 7*, 220–232 in press

Hargadine, JR, Branston, NM, Symon, L (1980). Central conduction time in primate brain ischaemia—A study in baboon. *Stroke, 11*, 637–642

Heiss, WD, Rosner, G (1983). Functional recovery of cortical neurons as related to degree and duration of ischemia. *Ann Neurol, 14*, 294–301

Hossman, KA, Kleihues, P (1973). Reversibility of ischemic brain damage. *Arch Neurol, 29*, 375–384

Jennett, B, Teasdale, G (1981). *Management of head injuries.* Philadelphia: FA Davis Company

Kaga, K, Hink, RE, Shinoda, Y, Suzuki, J (1980). Evidence for a primary cortical origin of the middle latency auditory evoked potential in cats. *Electroencephalogr Clin Neurophysiol, 50*, 242–266

Karnaze, DS, Marshall, LF, McCarthy, CS, et al. (1982). Localizing and prognostic value of auditory responses in coma after closed head injury. *Neurology, 32*, 299–302

Klug, N (1982). Brainstem auditory evoked potentials in syndromes of decerebration, the bulbar syndrome and in central death. *Neurol, 227*, 219–228

Kopf, GS, Hume, AL, Durkin, MA, et al. (1985). Measurement of central somatosensory conduction time in patients undergoing cardiopulmonary bypass: An index of neurologic function. *Am J Surg, 149*, 445–447

Korein, J (1980). Brain death. In JE Kottrel & H Turndorf (Eds.), *Anesthesiology in neurosurgery* (pp. 282–231). St. Louis: CV Mosby

Kraus, N, Ozdamar, O, Heydemann, PT, et al. (1984). Auditory brainstem responses in hydrocephalic patients. *Electroencephalogr Clin Neurophysiol, 59*, 310–331

Lee, YS, Lueder, H, Dinner, DS, et al. (1984). Recording of auditory evoked potentials in man using chronic subdural electrodes. *Brain, 107*, 115–131

Lesnick, JE, Michele, JJ, Simeone, FA, et al. (1984). Alteration of somatosensory evoked potentials in response to global ischemia. *J Neurosurg, 60*, 490–494

Levin, HS (1985). Outcome after head injury: General considerations and neurobehavioral recovery. In DP Becker & JT Povlishock (Eds.), *Central nervous system trauma status report* (pp. 281–289). Bethesda: NINCDS, NIH

Lindsay, KW, Carlin, J, Kennedy, I, et al. (1981). Evoked potentials in severe head injury—Analysis and relation to outcome. *J Neurol Neurosurg Psychiatry, 44*, 796–802

Lutschg, J, Pfenninger, J, Ludin, HP, Fassela, F (1983). Brain-stem auditory evoked potentials and early somatosensory evoked potentials in neurointensively treated comatose children. *Am J Dis Child, 137*, 421–426

Marsh, RR, Frewen, TC, Sutton, LN, Potsic, WP (1984). Resistance of the auditory brainstem response to high barbiturate blood levels. *Otolaryngol Head Neck Surg, 92*, 685–688

Marshall, LF, Smith, RW, Shapiro, HM (1979). The outcome with aggressive treatment in severe head injuries. Part I. The significance of intracranial pressure monitoring. *J Neurosurg, 50*, 20–25

Marshall, NK, Donchin, E (1981). Circadian variation in the latency of brainstem responses and its relation to body temperature. *Science, 212*, 356–358

McPherson, D, Blanks, J, Foltz, E (1984). Intracranial pressure effects on the auditory evoked responses in the rabbit: Preliminary report. *Neurosurgery, 14*, 161–166

Messick, JM, Newberg, LA, Nugent, M, Fanst, RJ (1985). Principles of neuroanesthesia for the nonneurosurgical patient with CNS pathophysiology. *Anesth Analg, 64*, 143–174

Miller, TD, Becker, DP, Ward, JD, et al. (1977). Significance of intracranial hypertension in severe head injury. *J Neurosurg, 47*, 503–516

Mjoen, S, Nordby, HC, Torvic, A (1983). Auditory evoked brainstem responses (ABR) in coma due to severe head trauma. *Acta Otolaryngol, 95*, 131–138

Nagao, S, Roccaforte, T, Moody, RA (1979). Acute intracranial hypertension and auditory brainstem responses. Part I. Changes in the auditory brainstem and somatosensory evoked responses in intracranial hypertension in cats. *J Neurosurg, 51*, 669–676

Nagao, S, Sunami, N, Tsutsui, T, et al. (1982). Serial observations of brain stem function by auditory brain stem responses in central transtentorial herniation. *Surg Neurol, 17*, 355–357

Nakagawa, Y, Ohtsuka, K, Tsuru, M, Nakamura, N (1984). Effects of mild hypercapnia on somatosensory evoked potentials in experimental cerebral ischemia. *Stroke, 15*, 275–278

Narayan, RK, Greenberg, RP, Miller, JD, et al. (1981). Improved confidence of outcome prediction in severe head injury. A comparative analysis of the clinical examination, multi-modality evoked potentials, CT scanning and intracranial pressure. *J Neurosurg, 54*, 751–752

Newlon, PG, Greenberg, RP, Hyatt, MS, et al. (1982). The dynamics of neuronal dysfunction and recovery following severe head injury assessed with serial multimodality evoked potentials. *J Neurosurg, 57*, 168–177

Newlon, RG, Greenberg, RP, Enas, GG, Becker, DP (1983). Effects of therapeutic pentobarbital coma on multimodality evoked potentials recorded from severely head-injured patients. *J Neurosurg, 12*, 613–619

Nordby, HK, Nesbakken, R (1984). The effect of high dose barbiturate decompression after severe head injury. A controlled clinical trial. *Acta Neurochir, 72*, 157–166

Nordby, HK, Gunnerod, N (1985). Epidural monitoring of the intracranial pressure in severe head injury characterized by non-localizing motor response. *Acta Neurochir, 74*, 21–26

Osborn, AG (1977). Diagnosis of descending transtentorial herniation by cranial computed tomography. *Radiology, 123*, 93–96

Piatt, JH, Jr, & Schiff, SJ (1984). High dose barbiturate therapy in neurosurgery and intensive care. *Neurosurgery, 15*, 427–444

Rao, N, Jellinek, HM, Harvey, RF, Flynn, MM (1984). Computerized tomography head scans as predictors of rehabilitation outcome. *Arch Phys Med Rehabil, 65*, 18–20

Rappaport, M, Hall, K, Hopkins, K, et al. (1978). Evoked brain potentials and disability in brain-damaged patients. *Arch Phys Med Rehabil, 58*, 333–338

Reilly, EL, Kondo, C, Brunberg, JA, Doty, DB (1978). Visual evoked potentials during hypothermia and prolonged circulatory arrest. *Electroencephalogr Clin Neurophysiol, 45,* 100–106

Rockoff, MA (1984). Brain resuscitation—Barbiturates and other anesthetic agents. *Semin Neurol, 4,* 408–411

Rosenberg, C, Wogensen, K, Starr, A (1984). Auditory brainstem and middle- and long-latency evoked potentials in coma. *Arch Neurol, 41,* 835–838

Rosenblum, SM, Ruth, RA, Gal, TJ (1985). Brainstem auditory evoked potential monitoring during profound hypothermia and circulatory arrest. *Ann Otol Rhinol Laryngol, 94,* 281–283

Russ, W, Kling, D, Loesevitz, A, Hempelman, G (1984). Effect of hypothermia on visual evoked potentials in humans. *Anesthesiology, 61,* 207–210

Samra, SK, Krutak-Krol, H, Pohorecki, R, Domino, EF (1985). Scopolamine, morphine and brain-stem auditory evoked potentials in awake monkeys. *Anesthesiology, 62,* 437–441

Sato, M, Pawlik, G, Umbach, C, Heiss, WD (1984). Comparative studies of regional CNS blood flow and evoked potentials in the cat. Effects of hypotensive ischemia on somatosensory evoked potentials in cerebral cortex and spinal cord. *Stroke, 15,* 97–101

Saul, TG, Decker, TB (1982). Effect of intracranial pressure monitoring and aggressive treatment in mortality in severe head injury. *J Neurosurg, 56,* 503–998

Seales, DM, Rossiter, VS, Weinstein, MD (1979). Brainstem auditory evoked responses in patients comatose as a result of blunt head trauma. *J Trauma, 19,* 347–353

Shapiro, K (1985). Head injury in children. In DP Becker & JT Povlishock (Eds.), Central nervous system trauma status report (pp. 243–253). Bethesda: NINCDS, NIH

Sklar, FH, Ehle, AL, Clark, WK (1979). Visual evoked potentials: A noninvasive technique to monitor patients with shunted hydrocephalus. *Neurosurgery, 4,* 529–534

Sohmer, H, Gafni, M, Chisin, R (1982). Auditory nerve-brain stem potentials in man and cat under hypoxic and hypercapnic conditions. *Electroencephalogr Clin Neurophysiol, 53,* 506–512

Sohmer, H, Gafni, M, Goitein, K, Fainmesser, P (1983). Auditory nerve brainstem evoked potentials in cat during manipulation of the cerebal perfusion pressure. *Electroencephalogr Clin Neurophysiol, 55,* 198–202

Sohmer, H, Gafni, M, Havatselet, G (1984). Persistence of auditory nerve response and absence of brain-stem response in severe cerebral ischaemia. *Electroencephalogr Clin Neurophysiol, 58,* 65–72

Stern, BJ, Krumholz, A, Weiss, HD, et al. (1982). Evaluation of brainstem stroke using brainstem auditory evoked responses. *Stroke, 13,* 705–711

Sutton, LN, Bruce, DA, Welsh, F (1980). The effects of cold-induced brain edema and white-matter ischemia on the somatosensory evoked response. *J Neurosurg, 53,* 180–184

Sutton, LN, Frewen, T, Marsh, R, et al. (1982). The effects of deep barbiturate coma on multimodality evoked potentials. *J Neurosurg, 57,* 178–185

Swann, KW (1984). Intracranial pressure monitoring devices. *Semin Neurol, 4,* 412–416

Taylor, MJ, Houston, BD, Lowry, NJ (1983). Recovery of auditory brain-stem responses after a severe hypoxic-ischemic insult. *N Engl J Med, 49,* 1169–1170

Teasdale, E, Cardoso, E, Galbraith, S, Teasdale, G (1984). CT scan in severe diffuse head injury: Physiological and clinical correlations. *J Neurol Neurosurg Psychiatry, 47,* 600–603

Toutant, SM, Klauber, MR, Marshall, LF, et al. (1984). Absent or compressed basal cisterns on first CT scan: Ominous predictors of outcome in severe head injury. *J Neurosurg, 61,* 691–694

Tsubokawa, T, Nishimoto, H, Yamamoto, T, Kitamura, M, Katayama, Y, Moriyasu, N. (1980). Assessment of brainstem damage by the auditory brainstem response in acute severe head injury. *J Neurol Neurosurg Psychiatry, 43,* 1005–1011

Umbach, C, Heiss, WD, Traupe, H (1981). Effect of graded ischemia on functional coupling and components of somatosensory evoked potentials. *J Cereb Blood Flow Metab, 1 (Suppl. 1),* s198–s199

Uziel, A, Benezech, J (1978). Auditory brainstem response in comatose patients. Relationship with brainstem responses and level of coma. *Electroencephalogr Clin Neurophysiol, 45,* 515–524

Van Dongen, KJ, Braakman, R, Gelpkel, GJ (1983). The prognostic value of computerized tomography in comatose head-injured patients. *J Neurosurg, 59,* 951–957

Ward, JD, Becker, DP, Miller, JD, Choi, SC, et al. (1985). Failure of prophylactic barbiturate coma in the treatment of severe head injury. *J Neurosurg, 62,* 383–388

Yagi, T, Baba, N (1983). Evaluation of the brain-stem function by the auditory brainstem response and the caloric vestibular reaction in comatose patients. *Arch Otorhinolaryngol, 238,* 33–43

York, DH, Pulliam, MW, Rosenfeld, JG, Watts, C (1981). Relationship between visual evoked potentials and intracranial pressure. *J Neurosurg, 55,* 909–916

Zimmerman, RA, Bilaniuk, LT, Gennarelli, TA (1978). Cranial computed tomography in diagnosis and management of acute head trauma. *Am J Roentgenol, 131,* 27–34

Zuccarello, M, Fiore, DL, Pardatscher, K, et al. (1983). Importance of auditory brainstem responses in the CT diagnosis of traumatic brainstem lesions. *Am J Neuroradiol, 4,* 481–483

Robert Aaron Levine

6

Surgical Monitoring Applications of the Brainstem Auditory Evoked Response and Electrocochleography

Short-latency auditory evoked potentials are becoming widely used for intraoperative monitoring of procedures that place at risk brainstem (pons to midbrain), auditory nerve, or cochlea, because the potentials provide rapid feedback about the physiologic state of a region of the nervous system that had been previously unassessable. The surgeon can now use these potentials to guide surgery. From our experience in monitoring surgery for cerebellopontine angle tumors, we have described some fundamental considerations in optimizing both the stimulus and recording systems. We show that recording the electrocochleogram (ECochG) along with the brainstem auditory evoked response (BAERs) has distinct advantages over recording the BAERs alone. Of all the components of the BAERs, wave I, the compound action potential of the auditory nerve, has by far the best predictive value for hearing outcome; the ECochG also records this potential (termed N-1). An advantage of the ECochG is that N-1 is typically about an order of magnitude larger than wave I. Another advantage of the ECochG is that, unlike the BAERs, which provide no information about the state of the cochlea, the ECochG routinely records a potential generated within the cochlea, the cochlear microphonic (CM). Not only is CM useful as a monitor of the state of the cochlea, but at times a change in CM is the first warning of a major hearing change.

Patterns of changes in the potentials are described, including direct evidence that sacrificing a blood vessel can disrupt auditory nerve and cochlea function. Clamping of blood vessels before cautery will predict the outcome of the cautery for the evoked potentials and will influence the decision about whether or not to sacrifice the blood vessel.

Finally, several artifactual changes in the potentials are pointed out. The value of monitoring the sound pressure in the external auditory canal for distinguishing between artifactual and real changes in the evoked potentials is stressed.

Most major neurosurgical procedures are done with general anesthesia. A major problem is that the patient cannot report on the functional status of the parts of his or her nervous system at risk from the procedure. Until recently, the only information generally available to the surgeon has been the gross anatomical state of the structures within the surgical field, and the patient's cardio-respiratory status. Since neurophysiologic activity is little affected by general anesthesia it can be used to alert the surgical team to physiologic changes that otherwise would go unnoticed. For example, spontaneous electroencephalographic activity has been used to detect cerebral ischemia that may occur during carotid artery surgery (Ojemann et al., 1975). Advances in miniaturization of noise reduction instruments has made it possible to monitor even smaller electrical signals, such as the sensory-evoked potentials (Levine et al., 1978).

Some properties of the short-latency auditory evoked potentials make them particularly well-suited for intraoperative monitoring. Like the short-latency potentials of other sensory modalities, these potentials are relatively resistant to anesthetics; unlike the other sensory modalities, these potentials change relatively little as the rate of stimulation is increased. Consequently, noise reduction (and signal detection) by signal averaging can be accomplished more rapidly with auditory evoked potentials, and so feedback about the physiologic status of the auditory pathway typically can be obtained in a few seconds.

The short-latency auditory evoked potentials can be recorded by two techniques: one near-field (the electrocochleogram or ECochG) and the other far-field (the brainstem auditory evoked responses or BAERs). These two techniques complement each other, since only the ECochG records potentials generated within the cochlea, while only the BAERs include potentials generated within the brainstem. These two techniques also overlap each other, since potentials generated by the auditory nerve are recorded by both the ECochG (as N-1) and the BAERs (as

Clinical Atlas of Auditory Evoked Potentials
ISBN 0-8089-1896-6

wave I). Because the sources of these potentials are within the 3 major sections of the lower auditory system (cochlea, auditory nerve, and brainstem), the ECochG and BAERs are well-suited for monitoring hearing during any surgery that might put any one of these sites at risk. One such surgery is cerebellopontine angle tumor removal. In patients who have some hearing beforehand, there has been a high incidence of hearing loss with surgery despite leaving the auditory structures grossly intact. Since 1977, we have been monitoring hearing during surgery of cerebellopontine tumors using ECochG and BAERs with two objectives in mind. The short-term objective is to help save the hearing of the patient being monitored by providing rapid feedback to the surgeon about any change in the patient's potentials. The surgeon can then either modify the approach to the tumor to minimize such changes, or can use other therapeutic maneuvers to improve the chance of saving the patient's hearing. Our long-term objective is to study the pattern of physiologic changes that occur in order to generate hypotheses about what might be the mechanism(s) of the hearing loss. From these hypotheses will follow ideas about what can be done differently to improve the

chance of saving hearing with surgery. In what follows, we will describe: (1) the techniques we have developed for intraoperative monitoring during surgical removal of cerebellopontine angle tumors; (2) some of the patterns of changes that have been observed; and (3) some of the pitfalls in interpreting the changes in these potentials.

RECORDING SYSTEM

Our recordings have all been made during the suboccipital, posterior fossa approach to cerebellopontine angle tumors, the vast majority of which have been acoustic neuromas (vestibular schwannomas), benign tumors that typically arise within the internal auditory canal and may spread into the cerebellopontine angle of the posterior fossa (Fig. 6-1). Our surgical team consists of a neurosurgeon, who exposes the cerebellopontine angle and removes the tumor within this region, and an otolaryngologist who opens the internal auditory canal and resects the tumor from within the canal.

Figure 6-1. Four different views of an acoustic neuroma. Panels A, B, and C are all from Subject 397, who had a 1.5-cm (maximum diameter) right-sided acoustic neuroma. In A, the arrow points to the acoustic neuroma (AN), as shown on the contrast-enhanced CT scan. In B, the arrows point to the right and left internal auditory canals (IAC) as they appear on a CT image that has been formatted to accentuate the boney landmarks. As shown on the right, frequently an AN will enlarge the IAC. The magnetic resonance image of panel C shows how the tumor may appear mushroom-shaped. The stalk is the image of the tumor within the IAC and the cap is the tumor within the cerebellopontine angle (between the brain and the temporal bone). Panel D is a photograph, taken through the operating microscope, of a 2.5-cm tumor from Subject 125. (R = retractors on cerebellum; T = tentorium; IAM = internal auditory meatus.)

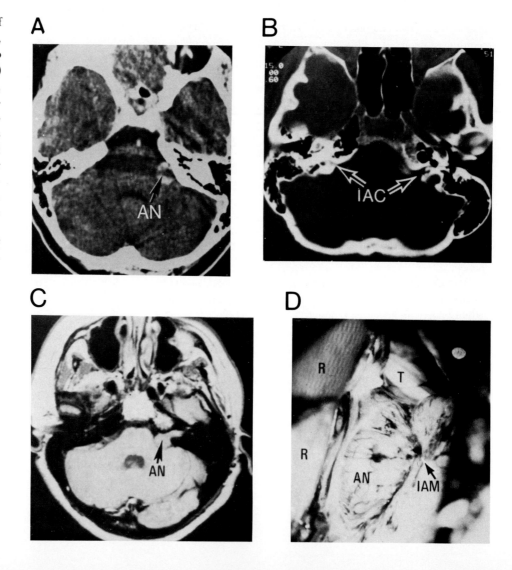

In Figure 6-2 is a block diagram of a system that is just adequate for intraoperative monitoring. The electrocochleogram and the brainstem auditory evoked potentials are recorded simultaneously on separate channels. For the ECochG, the active (positive) electrode is a needle electrode placed through the inferior part of the tympanic membrane to rest on the promontory of the medial wall of the middle ear. The only morbidity with this electrode has been, on one occasion, a tear in the tympanic membrane that repaired spontaneously. A needle electrode within the ipsilateral earlobe is used as the reference. At present, our most satisfactory transtympanic electrode has been constructed from a 3-inch, 29-guage, stainless steel hypodermic needle that has been insulated to within 4 mm of its tip by sliding over its shaft thin-walled Teflon tubing (internal diameter = .009 in). Because the size of the 2 components of the ECochG (cochlear microphonic and the compound action potential of the auditory nerve) can vary with the electrode position, the electrode may need repositioning to find a place where relatively large potentials can be obtained. Once final placement has been selected, the shaft is given a right-angle crimp at the level of the external auditory meatus and then taped securely to the side of the face, in such a way that the tip of the electrode remains under tension against the promontory of the middle ear (Fig. 6-3.).

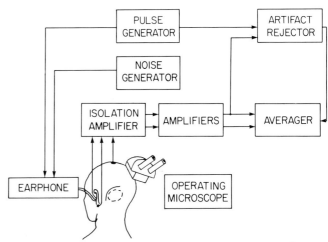

Figure 6-2.   Block diagram of a stimulus-generating and stimulus recording system that is just adequate for intraoperative monitoring.

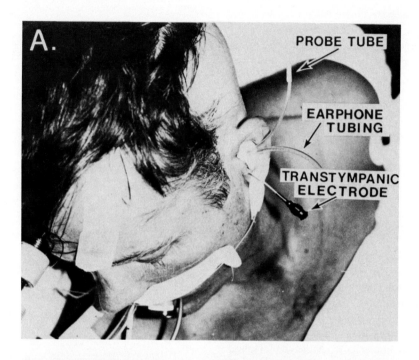

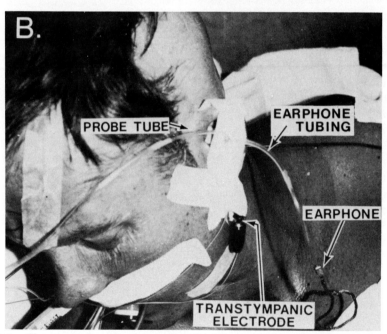

Figure 6-3.   The ear on the side of the tumor (A) following placement of the electrodes and custom-fit ear-mold, and (B) after attachment of the earphone and probe-tube microphone, and securing the ear-mold and transtympanic electrode with tape. The probe tube and earphone tubing pass through a hole in the center of the ear-mold. The transtympanic electrode does not pass through the ear-mold, but lies between the ear-mold and the ear canal. The probe tube microphone is not pictured.

The BAERs are recorded differentially between needle-electrodes near the vertex of the head and the ipsilateral earlobe or the nape of the neck. The first stage of amplification must be with an amplifier that is electrically isolated from the remainder of the system, so that significant current cannot pass between the equipment and the patient. Care must be taken to minimize the noise being picked up by the recording electrodes or their leads. The noise contribution of each piece of electrical equipment in the operating theater must be minimized. The leads should be kept as short as possible, and, when possible, the pair of leads to each differential amplifier should be twisted together, in order to keep the noise from these leads as small as possible. The first stage of amplification should have a fixed band width of about 1–3000Hz on all channels, and a gain of 100 or more. It is followed by a second stage of amplification with selectable gain and filters. For the ECochG, a high-pass cut-off of between 30 and 100Hz and a low pass cut-off of about 3000 Hz is usually desirable. For the BAERs a low pass cut-off of about 1000Hz usually provides good definition of the peaks while eliminating higher-frequency noise. The high-pass cut-off should be chosen with care. The BAERs generally consist of a single low-frequency peak of more than 5 msec duration, upon which are superimposed 5 or more high-frequency peaks of about 1 msec duration each (Levine, 1982). As shown in the BAERs of a normal subject in Figure 6-4, by setting the high-pass cut-off about 50Hz, the low-frequency component of the BAERs will be attenuated so that the overall size of the signal being monitored will be reduced. All other things being equal, the effect of the reduced signal size is to lengthen the time needed to detect the BAERs and provide feedback to the surgeon. Since in some patients with acoustic neuromas their high-frequency peaks are smaller than normal or even absent, while their low-frequency peak is relatively spared, attention to the high-pass cut-off will many times allow detection of a signal in the BAERs that might otherwise be filtered out (Levine, 1979). The exact choice of the high-pass cut-off will depend upon the filter characteristics of the system being used. Steeper filters and larger phase shifts than those shown in Figure 6-4 may require selecting an even lower cut-off. Each system should be individually evaluated.

The overall gain of the amplification system will depend upon the range of the analog-to-digital converter of the averaging system. In general, the gain should be set high enough so that the converter is occasional but rarely saturated, in the absence of artifacts (such as electrocautery).

When large electrical artifacts are generated by such devices as electrocautery units, facial nerve stimulators, or ultrasonic or laser dissectors, the recordings are dominated by these artifacts, so that it is always a better strategy to halt averaging and wait for the artifact to stop rather than to continue averaging. A component of the system that automatically recognizes an artifact (by such features as its large amplitude) and stops the averaging process not only makes the operation of the system much simpler, but also more efficient and accurate than is manual operation. One difficulty with most automated systems is related to the problem of blocking of the amplifiers. When an artifact becomes very large, it can cause an amplifier to "block." For several seconds after the artifact is over, there will be no output from the amplifiers, until there is a final return to normal

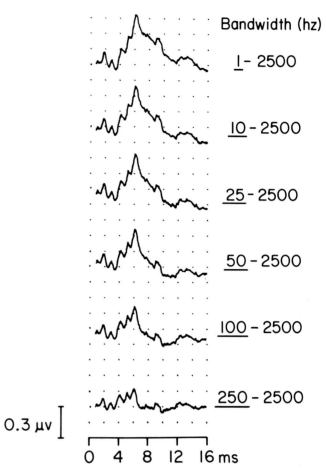

Figure 6-4. Effect of the high-pass cut-off on the BAERs. The BAERs of a normal subject are shown processed with 6 different settings of a 6-dB/octave high-pass filter. Notice that the maximum amplitude of the waveform decreases progressively for settings of 50Hz and above. Subject 8. Stimulus: 10/sec, monaural rarefaction clicks at 70 dB nHL. Electrodes: vertex(+), ipsilateral earlobe(−). In this and all figures, vertex positivity is plotted upward.

mode. Blocking can be readily recognized because the output of the amplifiers will appear markedly attenuated when viewed on an oscilloscope. Unless it is designed to detect blocking, an automatic artifact rejector will faithfully allow the average process to continue while the amplifiers are blocked. Consequently, initially, many sweeps may contain no signal, so that an averaged waveform may occur in which the response will appear small, not because there has been a change in hearing, but because for several of the sweeps contributing to the average no signal was present.

The averager sampling time ideally should be less than 125 μsec in order to faithfully reproduce CM. However, sampling times as long as 500 μsec are sufficient for recording the N-1 and BAERs. To include the BAERs under all circumstances, the averager should sweep for at least 12 msec following the click. By beginning its sweep about 5 msec before the presentation of the click, the first part of each averaged waveform provides an estimate of the background noise level of the waveform (Figs. 6-5, 6-6, and 6-7).

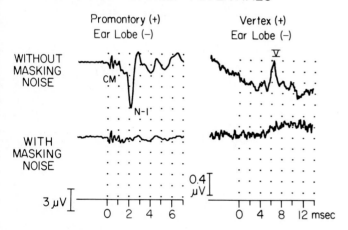

EFFECT OF MASKING NOISE ON AUDITORY EVOKED POTENTIALS

80 dB RC 33/sec, 75 dB SL Broadband Noise, Subject 242

Figure 6-5. ECochG and BAERs as recorded in response to clicks alone (top) and clicks mixed with broadband noise (bottom). In the presence of masking noise, both the N-1 and the BAERs become undetectable. Subject 242. Stimulus: 80 dB nHL, rarefaction clicks at 33/sec. Masking noise: 75 dB nHL broadband noise.

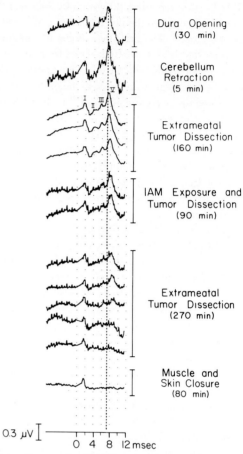

Figure 6-6. Successive BAERs recorded throughout the operation of subject 125. All the waves except wave I show a progressive loss in amplitude and increase in latency. No hearing was present postoperatively. Stimulus: 33/sec, condensation clicks at 80 dB nHL.

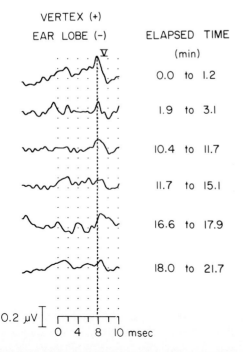

Figure 6-7. Loss of wave V amplitude and increase in its latency, as the tumor was dissected from the brainstem in the region of the eighth nerve. Some hearing was present postoperatively, but the speech discrimination score was 16 percent (down from 84 percent preoperatively). Subject 120. Stimulus: 45/sec, rarefaction clicks at 80 dB nHL.

The ECochG is generally of much larger amplitude than are the BAERs. In fact, many times wave I cannot be detected in the BAERs, and yet N-1 is easily detected in the ECochG (Figs. 6-5, 6-8, and 6-9). Many fewer trials need to be averaged for detecting the ECochG than for the BAERs; in a typical case, the ECochG may require about 50 trials and the BAERS about 1000 trials. Ideally, the averager should have the ability to accumulate the ECochG and BAERs independently for different numbers of trials so that they are both monitored near their limits of detectability. Otherwise, some compromise of monitoring both sets of potentials must be made. As will be elaborated later, if a choice must be made, monitoring the ECochG is preferable to monitoring the BAERs as an aid for hearing preservation during acoustic neuroma surgery.

When averaging is being done for monitoring purposes, a better approach is to use a method that is continually displaying a completed average. Once a number of trials have been averaged so that the desired degree of noise reduction has occurred,

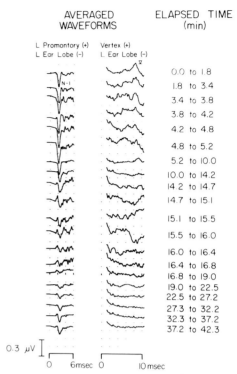

Figure 6-9. ECochGs and BAERs from subject 131 while her 1.5-cm tumor was being dissected off the eighth nerve complex. The BAERs abruptly disappear and are followed later by ECochG changes. The BAERs never reappeared during the operation, but the patient could hear postoperatively, nearly as well as preoperatively. Stimulus: 44/sec, condensation clicks at 78 dB nHL.

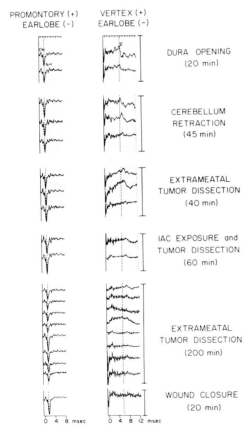

Figure 6-8. Representative ECochG and BAER waveforms obtained successively during complete removal of an acoustic neuroma (subject 406). The BAERs became progressively prolonged in latency and lowe in amplitude throughout the operation, so that by the time the tumor had been completely removed they were undetectable. In contrast, CM and N-1 were stable throughout. The patient's hearing was unchanged postoperatively. Compare to Figure 6-6. Stimulus: 29/sec, rarefaction clicks at 80 dB nHL.

rather than clearing the averager and starting again, the next trial is added to the average, while the first trial to contribute to the average is subtracted from the average. By repeating this procedure with each new trial, this "first in, first out" technique will always be displaying a completed waveform that is the average of the most recent trials. Exponential averaging is a similar technique that does not require a large memory capacity. It weights each trial, forming the average by a factor that becomes exponentially smaller in proportion to how many subsequent trials have occurred.

Two additional features of a monitoring system, while not essential, are desirable because they improve the efficiency of monitoring. These features are: (1) on-line plotting of the amplitude and latency of CM and N-1 of the ECochG and wave V of the BAERs, versus elapsed intraoperative time (such as shown in Figs. 6-10, 6-11, and 6-12); and (2) automatic clearing of the averager's memory and restarting of the averaging process after each average has been completed (for the systems that are not continually displaying a completed average).

Figure 6-10. Plot of N-1 and CM amplitudes obtained on-line over 8½ hours of the operation. Amplitudes were measured from the prestimulus baseline to peak of CM and N-1. Captions at left indicate the type of operative activity occurring over the period corresponding to the vertical bars. The bars with asterisks indicate intervals during which the wall of the internal auditory canal was being drilled. Waveforms on the right were obtained at the time to which the accompanying arrow points. N-1 is distinguished from CM by its sensitivity to masking noise. Papaverine was applied topically at the times marked by the short arrows and "P." Postoperatively, the patient's speech discrimination score was 56 percent (compared to 92 percent preoperatively), and his thresholds for 250 and 500Hz tones had worsened. Subject 268. Stimulus: 22/sec, rarefaction clicks at 80 dB nHL.

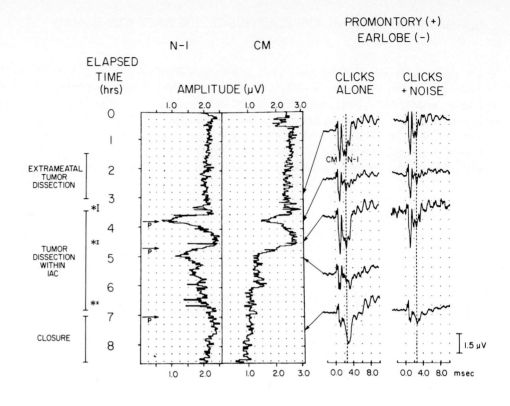

Figure 6-11. Plots of N-1 and CM amplitudes over 6 hours of operation with selected ECochGs. Note that at the beginning of the fourth hour, the first indication of a change in hearing is a growth in CM amplitude. It is then followed by loss of N-1 and postoperative hearing loss. The shaded portion of the bar during IAM exposure indicates the time when the dura over the IAM was being removed, and the unshaded portion indicates when the bone was being drilled. The patient had some detectable hearing during the first postoperative day, but none thereafter. Subject 233. Stimulus: 22/sec, rarefaction clicks at 80 dB nHL.

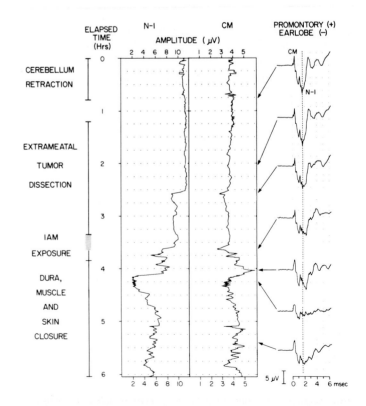

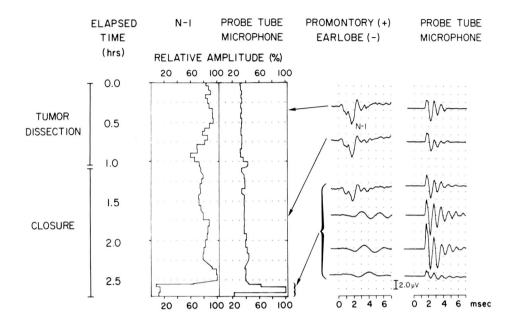

Figure 6-12. Plot of the amplitudes of the probe tube microphone recordings and N-1 over the last 2.5 hours of acoustic neuroma surgery (subject 396). These recordings were stable until the last 15 minutes. In this interval, the N-1 became very small and the probe tube recordings at first grew very large and finally very small. After the wound was closed, CSF was found welling up from the ear canal. CSF in the middle ear increases the impedance of the tympanic membrane, thereby increasing the size of the probe tube recordings. It also attenuates sound transmission through the middle ear, whereby, N-1 decreases. The final drop in the probe tube recordings was probably due to CSF entering the external ear canal and occluding the probe tube. Stimulus: 33/sec, rarefaction clicks at 70 dB nHL.

If the objective of monitoring is more than providing immediate feedback on the status of hearing, a more elaborate system with other features becomes desirable. In Figure 6-13 is a block diagram of one such system. The computer and disk provide a way of storing each waveform along with the time interval over which it was accumulated. The tape recorder preserves the analog signals before averaging, so that these signals may be analyzed again off-line with other averaging algorithms that would have been preferable for pinpointing the time of change in potentials. The video recorder preserves the surgical events as viewed through the operating microscope. Finally, the signal from the time-code generator marks the time the recordings were made on both the analog and video recorders, so that the physiological recordings and surgical events can be synchronized off-line, for reconstruction of the surgical events that led to a change in the potentials.

STIMULUS-GENERATING SYSTEM

The ideal stimulus for monitoring would be one that elicits as large a synchronous response as possible from as extensive a region of the cochlea and auditory pathway as possible. An earphone with a broad-band frequency response is desirable (the standard audiometric earphone is relatively narrow-band). Clicks are generally used as the stimulus, because they have a broad spectrum, short duration, and are readily generated by delivering an electric pulse to an earphone. Unfortunately, this pulse also produces an electrical signal that can be picked up by the recording electrodes and leads. This electrical artifact should be minimized by shielding the earphone and its cable, and by keeping the earphone and its cable far away from the recording electrodes and leads. If the artifact duration is long, it can overlap and obscure the earliest physiological responses. The most reliable method for distinguishing this artifact from the

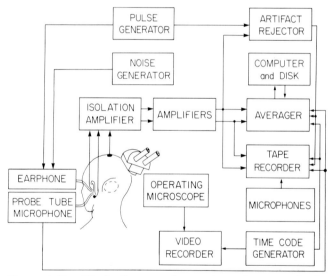

Figure 6-13. Block diagram of an enhanced system for intraoperative monitoring.

physiological responses is to separate them in time. In our present system, we create a 0.5-msec delay between the time the electrical signal arrives at the earphone and the time the click arrives at the ear. We use a Knowles ED-1932 receiver fitted into one end of a 6-inch polyvinyl tube (the first 3 inches of which is No. 16 tubing and the last 3 inches, No. 10 tubing) whose other end is positioned at the entrance to the ear canal in a custom-made ear mold (Figure 6-3).

Pulse duration affects the spectral content of the click, as well as the maximum level of any part of the spectrum. The shorter the pulse, the broader its band width, but the lower its maximum level. The limiting factor in the band width of the acoustic system will be the frequency response of the earphone. Generally, the pulse duration is shortened until the spectrum of the click no longer broadens. In our system, 60 μsec is the longest pulse duration before the click's band width narrows. The click level is usually set at the highest level possible by the system, since the potentials all grow monotonically with level (about 80 dB nHL, where 0 dB nHL = mean threshold of a group of normal hearing subjects). The other ear is masked by broad-band noise at about 40 dB nHL to prevent any BAERs due to acoustic cross-talk (Figure 6-14) (i.e., the clicks being presented to the operated ear are conducted to the other side and evoke BAERs from that ear).

For optimal monitoring of small signals, the signal-to-noise ratio per unit time (s:n/t) must be maximized. With higher click rates, 2 factors with opposite effects influence the s:n/t. On the one hand, with higher click rates, more trials can be completed per second so that the noise level of the average will be reduced more rapidly. On the other hand, our signals, the auditory evoked potentials, generally decrease in amplitude with higher click rates. It can be shown that the click rate that maximizes the function

$$(\text{peak amplitude}) \times \sqrt{(\text{rate})}$$

will be the optimum rate for monitoring, provided this rate corresponds to a period that is larger than the sweep time of the averager. As a general principle, since a major source of noise can be power line noise at a frequency of 60Hz (in the USA), the rate should be chosen so that it is not a sub-harmonic of this

frequency. In our experience, a rate near 30/sec is usually optimal. Because click polarity can also affect the amplitude of the BAER and N-1 of the ECochG, the response to both rarefaction and condensation clicks should be assessed for each patient and the one resulting in the larger amplitude response should be monitored (Fig. 6-15).

When a change occurs in our recordings, it is always possible that it is due to a failure somewhere in our stimulus-generating system. Because it is difficult to check out this possibility directly once the surgical drapes are in place, we use a probe tube system for quickly checking that the click arriving at the ear is unchanged. This system consists of a small hearing aid microphone (Knowles 1685) attached to one end of polyvinyl

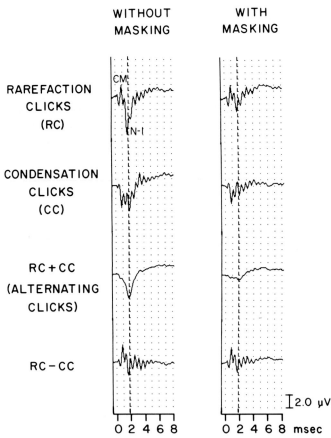

VERTEX (+)

IPSILATERAL EARLOBE (-)

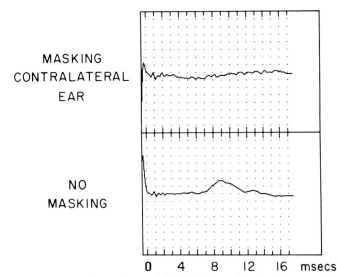

Figure 6-14. Recordings of the BAERs with and without masking of the contralateral ear. The peak at about 9 msec that occurs when there is no masking is due to acoustic cross-talk. Subject 408. Stimulus: 29/sec, condensation clicks at 80 dB nHL. Contralateral broadband masking at 30 dB nHL.

Figure 6-15. ECochG recordings to clicks alone and to clicks in the presence of a masking noise at about the same level as the click (80 dB nHL). CM is usually distinguished from N-1 by its greater resistance to masking and its ability to follow the polarity of the stimulus. The waveform recorded to alternating clicks will eliminate components of the ECochG that follow the phase of the click, whereas the difference waveform (RC − CC) waveform will eliminate components of the ECochG that do not change with reversing the click polarity. Subject 433. Click rate: 29/sec. Electrodes: promontory(+), ipsilateral earlobe(−). In this and all figures, promontory negativity is plotted downward.

tubing (No. 16) whose other end is at the entrance to the ear canal in the ear mold (Fig. 6-3). The signal from this microphone can be continuously monitored on an oscilloscope or can be incorporated into a third channel of the averaging system.

IDENTIFYING THE COMPONENTS OF THE EVOKED POTENTIALS

In Figure 6-5 are shown the ECochG and BAERs from a patient with relatively normal waveforms. We have been able to record the ECochG in all patients who have been monitored, for preservation of hearing, even when their speech discrimination scores were as low as zero. Two components of the ECochG can usually be identified: the cochlear microphonic and the compound action potential of the auditory nerve, the N-1, so called because it is normally the first major negative deflection in the ECochG. Two techniques can be used to distinguish these 2 components. First, the N-1 is more sensitive to masking noise than is the CM. Consequently, as shown in Figures 6-5 and 6-15, the addition of the masking noise virtually eliminates the first large negative component in the ECochG, thus confirming it as N-1. The second property that distinguishes these 2 components is demonstrated in Figure 6-15. The CM, as its name implies, behaves like a microphone and will follow a change in the click polarity, while the N-1, to a large extent, does not normally follow click polarity but remains a large negative component of the ECochG. Consequently, when the ECochGs for rarefaction and condensation clicks are compared, the component that changes polarity with the click polarity is likely to be the CM, while the component insensitive to click polarity is the N-1. Using alternating clicks to obtain a waveform (Fig. 6-15), or adding together the waveform obtained for rarefaction clicks with the waveform obtained for condensation clicks, will tend to cancel out the CM and leave behind the N-1. On the other hand, subtracting the waveforms for the 2 polarities will tend to eliminate N-1 and leave behind only the CM (Fig. 6-15). Use of these techniques may not be necessary when the typical ECochG appearance is seen in Figures 6-5 and 6-15, with the CM appearing as a high-frequency oscillatory response with very short

latency, and the N-1 as a larger, broader, later negative component. However, sometimes the ECochG does not have this typical appearance, and these 2 techniques must be relied upon for trying to distinguish these 2 components of the ECochG (Fig. 6-10).

Another property that is sometimes helpful in distinguishing CM from N-1 is their different sensitivities to click intensity. As the click level is increased from threshold, usually N-1 is the first component to appear and only at higher levels will the CM appear. When the stimulus artifact overlaps the ECochG, distinguishing the CM from the artifact may become difficult, since both follow the polarity of the stimulus and are relatively resistant to masking. The one property that can be used to distinguish the two is that CM can be at least partially masked with very high levels of noise (such as may occur with drilling the calvarium or temporal bone), while the stimulus artifact cannot be masked with any level of acoustical noise.

The BAERs are virtually always abnormal in these patients. In fact, this feature is used diagnostically to detect these tumors. In about 30 percent of our patients, no BAERs were detected (with the possible exception of wave I). Of the components of the BAERs, wave V is the largest and the one monitored; moreover, whenever it has been lost, waves II, III, and IV have always been lost as well. Wave I corresponds to N-1 of the ECochG, but is typically about an order of magnitude smaller than N-1 and sometimes cannot be detected at all in the presence of N-1. When present, however, it sometimes is useful as a check on N-1, should there be some question about whether or not changes in the ECochG are artifactual (Figs. 6-16 and 6-17). Masking the opposite ear will prevent recording any potentials generated by stimulating the uninvolved side (Fig. 6-14) with acoustic cross-talk.

PATTERNS OF CHANGE DURING SURGERY

During cerebellopontine angle tumor surgery, the auditory evoked potentials have shown several different patterns of change. The only pattern that has been consistently associated

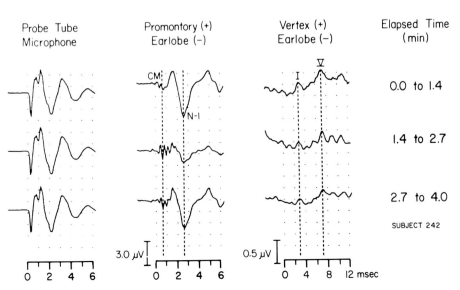

Figure 6-16. Simultaneous recordings of ECochG, BAER, and probe tube microphone. The striking alterations in CM and N-1, despite stable BAER and probe tube microphone recordings, suggest that these changes are due to fluctuations in the ECochG recording system, such as in promontory electrode contact. This same pattern recurred several times throughout the operation. Subject 242. Stimulus: 33/sec, condensation clicks at 80 dB nHL.

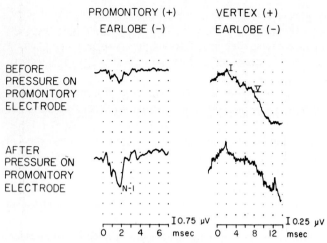

PROMONTORY (+)   VERTEX (+)
EARLOBE (-)   EARLOBE (-)

BEFORE
PRESSURE ON
PROMONTORY
ELECTRODE

AFTER
PRESSURE ON
PROMONTORY
ELECTRODE

N-1

I 0.75 µV   I 0.25 µV

0 2 4 6 msec   0 4 8 12 msec

Figure 6-17. Improvement of ECochG with putting pressure on the promontory electrode. Wave I of the BAERs shows little or no change, while the N-1 amplitude increases by more than a factor of three. Subject 396. Stimulus: 33/sec, rarefaction clicks at 70 dB nHL.

with no hearing change is when the BAERs and ECochGs remain unchanged throughout the operation. Once a change in these signals has occurred, then the degree of the hearing preservation cannot be reliably predicted. It may be well preserved, or there may be major changes. Even an apparent "improvement" in the evoked potentials, such as an increase in amplitude of N-1, may be associated with deterioration in the hearing. The persistence of an altered wave V of the BAERs does imply that some hearing will be preserved, but it does not predict its quality. A major improvement in hearing has never occurred in our patients following their tumor removal (Ojemann et al, 1984). These relationships between the changes in the evoked potentials and postoperative hearing are probably related to the fact that, in general, these evoked potentials are not reliable predictors of the quality of hearing (in terms of speech discrimination scores or pure-tone thresholds) in patients with cerebellopontine angle tumors as well as other disorders.

Wave V can change with or without changes in N-1. When changes occur *only* in wave V, they nearly always consist of a slowly progressive decline in amplitude and prolongation in latency. An abrupt change in only the BAERs rarely has been observed. Such changes are usually associated with changes in N-1 of the ECochG (Fig. 6-9) and are probably due to disruption of impulse generation in the auditory nerve at or before the generator site of N-1. Occasionally, small changes in wave V have been seen with cerebellar retraction (Fig. 6-8) and with dissection of the tumor from the brainstem (Fig. 6-7). The small size of the BAERs in most cases makes the detection of abrupt changes difficult. If we could detect the BAERs with the rapidity of the ECochG, we might find that some of the gradual losses are, in fact, a series of small, abrupt losses.

Loss of wave V (as well as all the other potentials following wave I) has poor predictive value for hearing outcome (Levine et

al., 1984; Friedman et al., 1985). When the loss is gradual, in some cases the hearing is lost (Fig. 6-6), and in other cases hearing is preserved (Fig. 6-8). When the loss is abrupt and associated with a transient loss in N-1, hearing may be preserved (Fig. 6-9).

N-1 and CM have proved to be more reliable than wave V for predicting whether some hearing will be preserved. If N-1 is lost by the end of the operation, then hearing has always been lost. If N-1 is present at closing, 90 percent of these patients will have some hearing; but about 10 percent will not (Fig. 6-6).

The changes in N-1 usually occur abruptly (Figs. 6-10, 6-11, and 6-18), but may sometimes be gradual, as when dissecting the tumor from within the internal auditory canal (Fig. 6-19).

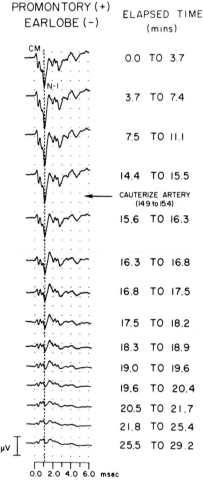

PROMONTORY (+)   ELAPSED TIME
EARLOBE (-)   (mins)

CM

N-1

0.0 TO 3.7

3.7 TO 7.4

7.5 TO 11.1

14.4 TO 15.5

CAUTERIZE ARTERY
(14.9 to 15.4)

15.6 TO 16.3

16.3 TO 16.8

16.8 TO 17.5

17.5 TO 18.2

18.3 TO 18.9

19.0 TO 19.6

19.6 TO 20.4

20.5 TO 21.7

21.8 TO 25.4

2.5 µV   25.5 TO 29.2

0.0 2.0 4.0 6.0 msec

Figure 6-18. Successive ECochGs from subject 356 as a small artery intimately involved with the last remaining piece of tumor was cauterized. To decide whether or not to sacrifice this blood vessel, it was first clamped for 20 sec. Because the ECochG remained unchanged, the vessel was then cauterized over 30 sec, during which time recordings could not be made. Immediately following cautery, the N-1 was already attenuated and then continued to disappear; slightly later, CM also became attenuated. Postoperatively the ear was deaf. These physiologic changes strongly suggest that this artery was the major blood supply for the cochlea. The BAERs were undetectable at the time of these recordings. Stimuli: 33/sec, rarefaction clicks at 70 dB nHL.

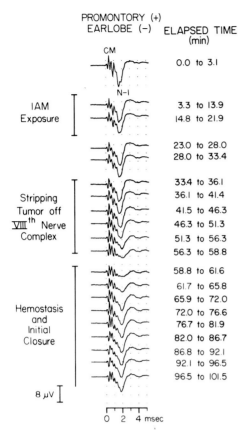

PROMONTORY (+)
EARLOBE (−) ELAPSED TIME
(min)

CM
0.0 to 3.1

N-1

IAM
Exposure
3.3 to 13.9
14.8 to 21.9

23.0 to 28.0
28.0 to 33.4

Stripping
Tumor off
VIIIth Nerve
Complex
33.4 to 36.1
36.1 to 41.4
41.5 to 46.3
46.3 to 51.3
51.3 to 56.3
56.3 to 58.8

Hemostasis
and
Initial
Closure
58.8 to 61.6
61.7 to 65.8
65.9 to 72.0
72.0 to 76.6
76.7 to 81.9
82.0 to 86.7
86.8 to 92.1
92.1 to 96.5
96.5 to 101.5

8 μV

0 2 4 msec

Figure 6-19. Gradual loss of N-1 but sparing of CM with dissection of 1-cm tumor out of internal auditory canal. Postoperatively, the patient's speech disrimination score was unchanged; pure-tone thresholds were poorer, at 4000 and 8000Hz. Subject 228. Stimulus: 22/sec, rarefaction clicks at 88 dB nHL.

Many times these changes are only transient (Figs. 6-9, 6-10, and 6-19). The N-1 changes are always associated with wave V alterations, but may occur with or without CM changes. On the other hand, CM changes are nearly always associated with N-1 changes. These patterns of relationships between inner ear (CM), auditory nerve (N-1), and brainstem (wave V) potentials fit with a simple sequential model that predicts that a change in one of these potentials will be associated with a change in all later potentials; but a change in a later potential can occur without any change in the earlier potentials.

Disturbances of the CM can appear as an increase (Fig. 6-11) or decrease (Fig. 6-10) in peak amplitude, as well as an overall change in its waveform (Fig. 6-11). This probably occurs because the CM is generated by cochlear hair cells, which are distributed in a complex geometric array. If the contribution from a section of the cochlea is reduced, it need not result in a loss in CM amplitude. Paradoxically, the CM amplitude could grow, if the activity from one part of the cochlea were cancelling out the contribution from another part of the cochlea. Because the cochlea itself is not directly in the field of this surgery, a disturbance of the CM suggests an indirect effect on the inner ear, such as compromising its blood supply (Levine et al., 1984). We now have direct evidence supporting this idea (Fig.

6-18). In fact, some of our operations suggest that the CM can sometimes be more sensitive to vascular changes than is the N-1; CM changes can precede N-1 changes (Fig. 6-11) and N-1 can appear to recover from an insult more fully than does the CM (Fig. 6-10).

On the basis of our observation that major changes in the ECochG can occur in the absence of any direct manipulations in the region of the tumor such as during wound closure (Ojemann et al., 1984), it is likely that alterations in the evoked potentials can occur after a delay from the time of the original insult. Vasospasm of the internal auditory artery is one mechanism that might account for these observations.

PITFALLS OF INTERPRETATION

A change in the pattern of evoked potentials is not always a sign that the patient's hearing has been altered. It sometimes may be due to extraneous factors involving either the stimulus or recording system. We have previously referred to an example due to the stimulus system: if the earphone suddenly fails, the evoked potentials will vanish abruptly. In our system, the loss of the signal from the probe tube microphone will immediately suggest this possibility. It can be confirmed by listening under the drapes for the stimulus, if the earphone is accessible.

Changes in the output from the probe tube microphone always suggest that alterations in the evoked potentials are due to an extraneous factor involving the stimulus system. One pattern has been observed several times. As the wound is being closed, the evoked potentials become attenuated and undergo major changes in configuration as the signal from the probe tube microphone grows in size (Fig. 6-12). When the ear is examined immediately following surgery, cerebrospinal fluid (CSF) has been found leaking into the middle ear and ear canal (through the puncture site of the transtympanic electrode). This occurs because mastoid air cells are sometimes entered with drilling of the skull or internal auditory canal. If the opening had not been adequately sealed with bone wax, once CSF pressure builds up with closure of the wound, CSF can leak into the middle ear.

Entering a mastoid air cell as the calvarium or internal auditory canal is being opened may also cause an immediate change in the evoked potentials. Simultaneous changes in the probe tube microphone recordings and the evoked potentials are the tipoff in these cases (Fig. 6-20).

Another major group of artifactual changes may occur due to difficulties with the recording system. The effect of blocking of the amplifiers has been mentioned earlier. In general, the signal will be lost when the recording system malfunctions. Putting a calibration signal at the input to the preamplifiers will test everything but the recording electrodes. A major increase in electrode impedance (from 5 kohm or less) will usually indicate a change in electrode contact (e.g., a dislodged scalp electrode). One exception to this generalization involves the transtympanic electrode, whose tip contacts the promontory of the middle ear. Typically, its impedance measures between 20 and 50 kohm. In Figure 6-16 are recordings from a case showing changes in both the N-1 and CM of the ECochG, while the probe tube monitor and the BAERs (including wave I) are perfectly stable. Because

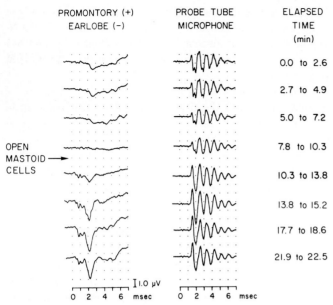

PROMONTORY (+)   PROBE TUBE   ELAPSED
EARLOBE (-)   MICROPHONE   TIME
                                            (min)

                                            0.0 to 2.6

                                            2.7 to 4.9

                                            5.0 to 7.2

OPEN   7.8 to 10.3
MASTOID →
CELLS   10.3 to 13.8

                                            13.8 to 15.2

                                            17.7 to 18.6

                                            21.9 to 22.5

                        ⊺ 1.0 µV

0 2 4 6 msec   0 2 4 6 msec

Figure 6-20. Successive ECochG and probe tube microphone recordings during a 22-minute interval that included opening of mastoid air cells in the process of drilling away the posterior wall of the internal auditory canal. Both the ECochG and the probe tube recordings increased at the time the air cells were opened. This association strongly links the changes in the potentials to the acoustical changes, even though the mechanism is not apparent. Subject 362. Stimulus: 33/sec, rarefaction clicks at 70 dB nHL.

wave I of the BAERs of the ECochG have the same generator, the changes in N-1 of the ECochG must be due to an extraneous factor. Since it has been shown that small changes in the position of a promontory electrode can sometimes result in large changes in configuration of the ECochG recordings (Montandon et al., 1975), it is likely that these ECochG changes are due to changes in the transtympanic electrode contact, despite no change in the measured electrode impedance.

A more dramatic and common example is shown in Figure 6-17. The ECochG had diminished to a barely detectable level; by putting pressure on the electrode near the earmold, the ECochG amplitudes immediately were restored, despite little or no change in the BAERs or the electrode impedance. The explanation for these observations appears to relate to electrode contact. By putting pressure on the promontory electrode, the contact at its tip is improved. The lack of a major change in electrode impedance needs an explanation: it probably is related to the construction of our electrode. The insulation of the elec-

trode stops about 4 mm from its tip, so that the contact of the uninsulated shaft with the tympanic membrane acts as a shunt resistance that dominates the total resistance of the electrode. This has recently been confirmed by using an electrode fully insulated down to the tip. This electrode's impedance decreases when the signal improves with putting pressure on the electrode.

Finally, extraneous sounds can alter the potentials and lead to misinterpretations. The problem of acoustic cross-talk has already been discussed. Background sounds can act as maskers, and, thereby, attenuate the evoked potentials (Figs. 6-5 and 6-15). In our experience, only the noise generated by drilling the skull has been intense enough to mask the potentials. Occasionally, the potentials will remain attenuated for several seconds following the drilling. This probably represents the phenomenon of temporary threshold shift.

ACKNOWLEDGMENTS

It is a pleasure to acknowledge the surgeons (Drs. R. Ojemann, W. Montgomery, R. Martuza, and J. Nadol), as well as the neuroanesthesia and operating room staffs. Thanks are due P. Riley for preparation of figures, Dr. S. Ronner for reviewing the chapter, and Dr. N. Kiang for his consistent support. This work was supported in part by U.S. Public Health Service Grant 5Po1 NS 13126.

REFERENCES

Friedman, WA, Kaplan, BJ, Gravenstein, D, Rhoton, AL (1985). Intraoperative brain-stem auditory evoked potentials during posterior fossa microvascular decompression. *J Neurosurg, 62*, 552–557

Levine, RA, Montgomery, WW, Ojemann, RG, Springer, MFB. (1978). Evoked potential detection of hearing loss during acoustic neuroma surgery. *Neurology 28*, 339

Levine, RA (1979). Monitoring auditory evoked potentials during acoustic neuroma surgery. In H Silverstein, & H Norrell (Eds.), *Neurological surgery of the ear*, vol. 2 (pp. 287–293). Birmingham, AL: Aesculapius Publishing

Levine, RA (1982). Auditory evoked potentials: Engineering considerations. *Proceedings of the fourth annual conference of IEEE; Engineering in medicine and biology society*, 85–88

Levine, RA, Ojemann, RG, Montgomery, WW, McGaffigan, PM. (1984). Monitoring auditory evoked potentials during acoustic neuroma surgery: Insights into the mechanism of the hearing loss. *Ann Otol Rhinol Laryngol, 93*, 116–123

Montandon, PB, Megill, ND, Kahn, AR, Peake, WT, Kiang, NYS (1975). Recording auditory-nerve potentials as an office procedure. *Ann Otol Rhinol Laryngol, 84*, 2–10

Ojemann, RG, Crowell, RM, Roberson, GH, Fisher, CM (1975). Surgical treatment of extracranial carotid occlusive disease. *Clin Neurosurg, 22*, 214–263

Ojemann, RG, Levine, RA, Montgomery, WW, McGaffigan, PM (1984). Use of interoperative auditory-evoked potentials when attempting to preserve hearing during removal of unilateral acoustic neuromas. *J Neurosurg, 61*, 938–948

Index

ABR. *See* Brainstem auditory evoked response (BAER)
Acoustic neuroma
   audiologic findings, 44t
   BAER, 43–44
      application in ruling out neuroma, 48f
      interpretation of, 33
      case study of, 10f, 44–47f
Action potential
   "compound", 2–3
   normal, 6t
   "whole-nerve", 2
Age
   maturational changes of BAER and, 63–64, 65t
   normal BAER and, 31t
AP. *See* Action potential
Artifacts
   amplifier blocking and, 107
   in BAER, 74
   during intraoperative monitoring, 107
   in stimulus-generated systems, 111
   and value of ECochG/BAER monitoring, 103
Audiograms, abnormal responses in, 6f
Auditory brainstem response. *See* Brainstem auditory evoked response (BAER)
Auditory evoked response. *See specific auditory evoked response*
Auditory middle-latency response (AMR)
   acquisition parameters, t
   advantages and disadvantages of, 19
   cognitive/communicative outcome in brain injury and, 97–98f
Auditory nerve action potential
   "compound", 2–3
   description of, 2–3
   "whole-nerve", 2
Auditory stimulus-related responses, in electrocochleography (ECochG), 2–3

BAEP. *See* Brainstem auditory evoked response

BAER. *See* Brainstem auditory evoked response
Barbiturates, evoked responses and, 77f
Bilateral hearing loss, case study of, 7–8f
Brain death determination
   BAER and, 49–50
   case studies
      of adults, 50–51f, 93–96f, 95f
      of children, 68–70f, 96f
   definition criteria, 93
   SSER and, 50
Brain injury, acute
   brain death determination. *See* Brain death determination
   CNS assessment criteria, 73
   factors influencing evoked responses in ICU
      artifacts in ABR measurement, 74
      body temperature, 75–77f
      otologic pathology, 74–75f
      therapeutic modalities, 77f
   neuroradiology, 83–92f
   prediction of cognitive/communicative outcome, 97–99f
   relationships among ABR and other findings, 78–83f
   SER and, 100
Brainstem
   glioma, 56f, 67
   infarction, 57f
   parenchymal lesions, 55–59f
   tumors, 58f, 59f. *See also specific tumors*
Brainstem auditory evoked response (BAER)
   abnormal, with normal pupils in adult, 81f
   for acoustic neuromas, 43–47f
   acquisition parameters of, 30t
   advantages of, 15–16
   age and, 31t
   amplitude of, 20, 33
   in assessment of pediatric hearing loss, 70f

case studies, 20–28f
   of cerebellopontine angle lesion not associated with eight nerve, 49f
   of cerebral death determination, 50–51f
   of coma following hypoxic-ischemic cerebral injury, 55f
   of conductive hearing loss, 37f
   of pontine hemorrhage, 54f
   of prolonged coma following cerebral trauma, case study, 52–53f
   of sensorineural hearing loss, 38f
click-elicited
   acquisition parameters of, 19t
   case studies of, 20–28f
   normative latency of, 19t
in comatose state, 49–50
disadvantages of, 16
hearing aid recommendation and, 20
high-frequency hearing loss effects, 38
intraoperative monitoring with ECochG, 103
   recording system, 104–111f
   stimulus-generating system, 111–113f
latency
   absolute, 30t
   interpeak, 30t, 34t
   normative values, 18t, 19t
maturation and norms, 63–64, 65t
in meningitis, 66–67
in multiple sclerosis, 38–39
of neonates and children
   in intensive care unit, 65–66
   technical factors in intrepretation and recording, 64–65
in neonates and young children, 63, 64f
in neurodegenerative disease, 68, 69f
and neurodiagnostic findings, 79–82f
neurologic applications
   multiple sclerosis, 40–42f
   pediatric, 63–70f, 70–71
neurologic applications, 29. *See also specific neurologic disorder*

117